A Survey
of Communication Disorders
for the Classroom Teacher

Martha Scott Lue

University of Central Florida

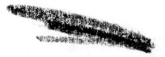

Allyn and Bacon

Boston • *London* • *Toronto* • *Sydney* • *Tokyo* • *Singapore*

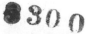

In appreciation, respect, and gratitude to my parents, Solomon and Rachel Scott, who, over fifty years ago, planted a seed that sprouted the belief that I could be anything that I wanted to be; and to my son, Marvin Charles Lue, Jr., whose grand entrance into my life over twenty-eight years ago continues to remind me of the awesomeness of God's presence

Editor in Chief: *Paul A. Smith*
Executive Editor and Publisher: *Stephen D. Dragin*
Editorial Assistant: *Barbara Strickland*
Marketing Manager: *Brad Parkins*
Editorial Production Service: *Chestnut Hill Enterprises, Inc.*
Manufacturing Buyer: *Chris Marson*
Cover Administrator: *Brian Gogolin*
Electronic Composition: *Omegatype Typography, Inc.*

Copyright © 2001 by Allyn & Bacon
A Pearson Education Company
160 Gould Street
Needham Heights, MA 02494

Internet: www.abacon.com

Between the time Website information is gathered and published, some sites may have closed. Also, the transcription of URLs can result in typographical errors. The publisher would appreciate notification where these occur so that they may be corrected in subsequent editions.

Library of Congress Cataloging-in-Publication Data
Lue, Martha Scott.
     A survey of communication disorders for the classroom teacher / Martha Scott Lue.
          p.   cm.
     Includes bibliographical references and index.
     ISBN 0-205-30804-X
     1. Handicapped children—Education—United States.   2. Language arts—Remedial teaching—United States.   3. Speech disorders in children—United States.   4. Communicative disorders in children—United States.   I. Title.

LC4028 .L84 2001
371.91'4—dc21   00-057620

Printed in the United States of America

10 9 8 7 6 5 4 3 2   05 04 03 02

Contents

8 *Problems of Voice and Fluency: Identification and Remediation*   **137**

Preface

Communication in its highest form represents the single most identifying act that separates human beings from other species. The process of human communication represents an unparalleled tapestry of information woven by the brain from stimuli of movement, expression, and vocalization of the speaker. Researchers note that it is these communication forms that convey information with specificity and detail.

For both partners in communication, the sender and receiver, the act of communication depends on the anatomical structure of sensory organs, the physiological functioning of those structures, as well as genetic and environmental factors. Most individuals develop communication processes in a predictable, orderly, and sequential manner. But for some, communication breaks down, due in part to problems involving hearing, articulation, language, or fluency. The field of communication disorders studies these complex and involved problems.

Effective communication is an essential skill for all humans. Students with disabilities in the area of communication account for one-fifth of the students currently receiving services in special education. This fact, as well as the fact that most students with disabilities in the area of communication receive services from special and regular education teachers, makes it imperative for increased knowledge of pathology and of strategies to remediate.

In an introductory text, it is impossible to acquaint the reader with all there is to know about this discipline. However, suggested strategies and detailed bibliographies are provided to assist the reader in gaining clarity in the usefulness of this book. We hope that people using it will be motivated to continue their studies in communication disorders.

Acknowledgments

I have learned a lot about journeys since I began writing this book. While it is true that each journey starts with a single step, I hasten to add that all of these steps are not necessarily forward steps. We meet a lot of people along the way who help us to maintain our stride and propel us in displaying all of those positive attributes that our parents felt we held within ourselves.

The journey for me began in Monticello, Florida, the last child of the late Solomon and Rachel Scott. My parents loved all of us, four sisters and one brother, but I think that there was some special love for me—both from my father and mother. As far back as I can remember, my parents told me, Martha Yvonne, you are going to be somebody when you grow up! Throughout my years, when I've needed to find that special reservoir for support, I needed that statement! My sisters, Mary Helen, Naomi, and Annie Ruth, have helped to keep this dream alive. For them, I shall be forever grateful. My deceased brother, Solomon, Jr., who had a wonderful sense of humor, always enjoyed listening to me read. I miss that. My oldest nephew, Charles Edward Scott, who is more like a son, continues to love me unconditionally. My brother-in-law, Horace Eugene Simon, who entered our lives the same month my brother died, is so special in my family's life.

My elementary and high school teachers saw that something, too, that I did not see. A tall, slender, gangly child, with big eyes and hard-to-comb hair, my parents spent time on me, teaching me, telling me, and then they left it up to my teachers to extend the teaching and reinforce good citizenship. Ms. Rosa Lee Sloan, Sunday School Superintendent and elementary teacher, played a special role in motivating me. Willie Ree Williams, my high school speech and drama teacher, taught me the beauty of the spoken and written word. Dr. Marcus Boulware, Professor of speech-language pathology at Florida A & M University, helped me to secure scholarships to universities and places I only dreamed I could attend. To the faculty and staff in the College of Education, past and present, and especially to my colleagues in the program area of exceptional education, I owe a special note of gratitude.

My church family, Carter Tabernacle CME Church, Orlando, Florida, Rev. Roderick Zak, Pastor, serve as my extended family. Delta Sigma Theta Sorority, Orlando Alumnae Chapter, State of Florida, the Bahamas, and the Southern Region encouraged me along this journey. Nannette McLain and Thelma Dudley, who believed in this project, even during its infancy, and who can probably recite some of the lines of the vignettes, word for word, I thank you for your commitment and belief in me.

Jeanice Midgett started the writing journey with us, but who retired after over thirty years in the teaching profession, continued to motivate, encourage, and inspire me. To the contributing writers of specific chapters, Gwendolyn Alexander, Lee Cross, and Mary Little, thank you for your contributions and patience.

Special thanks to the student assistants, too numerous to mention, especially, Gwendolyn Ellison, Kori Moore, Sonya Conover, Sonja Gilliam, Karla Martin, Vonya Knighton, Bertha Gant, Derese Schakelford, Keva Miller, Mark Nealy, Purvie Patel, Robin Capers, Gloria White, and Alisha Kahn, who gave of their time and effort to help to shape this effort.

Steve Dragin, my Executive Editor, who believed that this project was special, and deserved a wider audience, I shall be eternally grateful for your confidence. Thanks to Myrna Breskin, the production editor, who inspired us to present the very best work that we could, in a timely and professional manner.

The following reviewers, whose comments and suggestions were so very helpful and enlightening, provided special help: Diane Andrew, Valdosta State University; Donald K. Cadley, Ashland University; and James Cantrell, Tennessee State University.

And to the many preservice and graduate students who have shared their stories, their dreams, their hopes in that everyone student should have an effective teacher, one who communicates effectively, and one who challenges them to communicate, in a mode that's appropriate, effective, and truly theirs,

I thank each of you for the JOURNEY

1

Language, Speech, and Communication: An Overview

Martha S. Lue and Mary Little

Chapter Objectives _____

On completion of this chapter, the reader will be able to:

- Compare and contrast the characteristics of communication, language, and speech;
- Discuss the legal foundations and changing roles for special education teachers; and
- Overview the contents of this textbook.

- Five-year-old Matthew was evaluated by the Preschool Evaluation Team. He presented with an intelligence quotient (IQ) in the moderate range. The child was not able to talk in one-, two-, or three-word sentences. His only recognizable utterance was "mommie." He is able to imitate the behaviors of other youngsters in his class, e.g., clapping his hands along with their clapping. The child has an attention span of less than five minutes and exhibits only very basic skills. Initially diagnosed as developmentally delayed, followed by trainable mentally handicapped, the child's current placement is in a class labeled as "varying exceptionalities." Both the speech pathologist and the special educator work very closely to create language activities to improve the child's communication skills.

- Four-year-old Jacob, a child with Down syndrome, was evaluated at the beginning of the school year and found to be developmentally delayed. He exhibited a short attention span and very low language skills. His Individualized Education Program goals included working on attention span and working on semantics and syntax. The speech-language pathologist and the special educator work collaboratively with all of the students in the class by coteaching a language class three times a week, right in the child's classroom.

- Amanda was very bubbly at birth. Her parents noticed, however, that the older she became, the fewer sounds she made. Amanda was given a hearing test at age six months and was found to have a sensorineural hearing loss. She was placed in an early intervention program for youngsters with hearing impairments and receives speech-language therapy on a daily basis.

Disorders of communication presented by *Matthew, Jacob,* and *Amanda* provide illustrations of the challenges that teachers in inclusive classrooms face daily. Further, they illustrate some of the various types of speech, language, and communication problems found in schools today. Given the continual changes in education for individuals with disabilities, especially as more students with special needs are educated in regular education settings, and the emergence of educational trends such as inclusive schooling, whole language, and collaborative teaching (Owens, 1999), it is imperative that future special and regular educators, as well as other professionals, be provided an opportunity to learn effective strategies in working with individuals with communication disorders, and how to implement these strategies in the classroom and in collaborative settings that include parents and other professionals.

The intent of this text is to assist the classroom teacher, direct service provider, or other professional in the understanding, identification, and remediation (as part of a collaborative team as well as in the classroom) of communication disorders in children and adolescents. We have chosen to concentrate on children and adolescents, rather than adults, because of the complexity of language problems that children and adolescents exhibit, and, as explained by Owens (1999), adults with language problems present an even more diverse group; therefore, it is outside the scope of this text to address these issues.

While meeting the specific prescriptive remediation needs of children and adolescents with communication disorders remains the primary responsibility of the speech-language professional, a shared responsibility in identifying, understanding, and assisting these individuals resides with the classroom teacher or direct service provider and other members of the education team.

As a matter of fact, it has been reported that approximately three-fourths of all children and adolescents with disabilities receive all or most of their education in a general education classroom. With this in mind, it is imperative that all teachers be aware of and assume the tremendous responsibility and opportunity for providing appropriate instruction (Mastropieri & Scruggs, 2000). For the child identified as having a communication disorder, slightly more than 87 percent are served in regular classes; 7.6 percent are seen in resource rooms; while 4.5 percent are served in separate classes (Kirk, Gallagher, & Anastasiow, 2000).

Lastly, the ability to effectively communicate is one of the most important aspects of an individual's development, and, indeed, should be of paramount concern for all educators at all levels across various curricula. It is hoped that, through this text, readers will gain a better understanding of the complexity as well as the wide range of problems affecting communication, language, and speech, and the critical role that each professional must play in providing an appropriate educational communication environment for all students.

Keep in mind that, in the classroom, a variety of students may be present who do not speak at all and require assistive/augmentative communication, students who must learn to read lips and operate assistive listening devices, as well as students who display socially inappropriate verbal and nonverbal communication skills in different situations. An understanding of these disabilities, as well as the ability to identify and refer individuals with these disabilities, is critical to collaborative, inclusive teaching. Perhaps Van Riper & Erickson (1996) summarized it best, addressing why a course in communication disorders is important for classroom teachers or the need for such a text:

> [W]e are delighted to be your guides because we know that those who have been deprived of the most fundamental of all human traits, the ability to communicate, need all the help and understanding they can get. (p. 2)

Reflection

- **Discuss personal accounts of people you know with disabilities in the areas of communication, language, and speech.**
- **Discuss the impact of disabilities in the areas of communication, language, and speech.**

This introductory chapter explores basic terms of communication, language, and speech. Components within each of these broad areas will be discussed, as well as the changing roles of special educators and classroom teachers in addressing the needs of students with disabilities in each area. Outlines of the remaining chapters of this book will be presented at the end of this chapter.

Communication

Communication is generally defined as the transmission and reception of information and knowledge among participants (Owens, 1994). It represents a basic need and function of humans (Heward, 2000; Owens, 1994) and typically uses multiple forms. An active process, it requires at least the sender who encodes the message, and the receiver who decodes the message.

Many factors can alter the effectiveness of communication. Communication has paralinguistic cues for intonation and emphasis, and nonlinguistic cues, including facial expressions, gestures, intonation, and movements that may serve to expand or distort the code. The skills involved are not ends in themselves, but means or instruments that must be placed at the service of helping outcomes in order to be meaningful. In humans, the development of communication, language, and speech overlap to some degree. The term *communicative competence* is attributed to Hymes (1974), a sociolinguist who has been important in describing and stressing the importance of the role of situational factors in communication. To effectively communicate, our communication competence includes how to interact, how to interact appropriately with one another within various social situations, and how to make sense of what others say and do in communication situations. Communication encompasses almost all interpersonal interactions—verbal and nonverbal.

Communication can be further refined into interindividual and intraindividual communication. Interindividual communication takes place between two or more people without restriction to live dialogue. Therefore, conversations between friends, whether in person, on television or film, or within the written communication of a letter, are all examples of this type of interindividual communication. Intraindividual communication occurs within one person who serves as both the sender and the receiver of the message; planning, self-regulating, meditating, and

Communication

Components of communication using speech and language, as well as communication behaviors lacking speech and language (e.g., tapping on a friend's shoulder) and those lacking speech (e.g., a written note.)

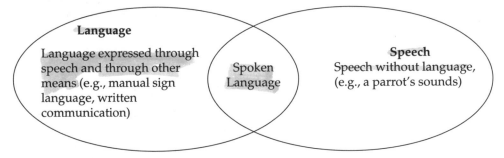

FIGURE 1.1 *Development of Communication, Language, and Speech*

From M. Hardman, C. Drew, & M. Egan. Human exceptionality (6th ed.). Copyright © 1999 by Allyn & Bacon.

feedback are examples. Thomas and Carmack (1990) noted that these types of messages occur constantly in our daily lives:

> Should I continue reading this chapter or go to the mall?
> Do I order a baked potato or French fries?
> I wonder how my friend will feel if I don't invite her to go?

Within daily communication, however, there can be differences noted that are not disorders. The American Speech-Language-Hearing Association defines communicative variations (ASHA, 1982): A **communicative difference** or **dialect** is a variation of the symbol system used by a group of individuals that reflects a shared regional, social, or cultural–ethnic factors. Owens (1988) adds that a dialect is a "language rule system of an identifiable group that varies from the rule system of an ideal standard" (p. 451). Variations or alterations in the use of the symbol system may be indicative of primary language interferences. A regional, social, or cultural–ethnic variation of a symbol system should not be considered a disorder of speech or language.

The term **augmentative communication,** in a general sense, refers to techniques and devices used by individuals to supplement whatever degree of naturally acquired speech they possess (Turnbull, Turnbull, Shank, & Leal, 1999). Both issues of communicative variations will be further explored in greater definition and detail in later chapters of this book.

Components of Communication

Communication has at least three components: a sender, a message, and a receiver. People can be the senders and receivers at the same time because they are both initiating communication and receiving the other's responses simultaneously. The message is the idea or thought being transmitted through the act of communication.

Morsink, Thomas, and Correa (1991) offered additional elements of the communication process:

- Channel is the route traveled by the message. This typically involves both sound and sight, because words are offered within a social contact involving nonverbal cues (e.g., facial expression, gestures, etc.)
- Feedback is the response of the senders and receivers to each other during the interaction. Feedback enables the sender to gauge whether or not the receiver understood the message as it was intended.
- Noise refers to the physical or psychological interference that may possibly prevent the message from being accurately comprehended.
- Setting is the location where the communication is taking place. It may be either formal or informal. The setting can impact the feelings people have while they are communicating.

Activities

• In pairs, one partner tells a short incident to his or her partner about something that happened during the last week that was very important or exciting. As the partner receiving the information, provide no verbal or nonverbal feedback. What happens? How does the speaker react? How does the speaker feel? Why do you think this happened?

• Think about three very different settings that you have visited during the last week (i.e., the mall, the movies, a football game, etc.). Discuss how the setting impacted the type of communication and feelings you had while you were in the various settings.

Components of Nonverbal Communication

Nonverbal communication refers to the nonverbal behaviors and mannerisms that may or may not accompany the verbal message in social interactions. Nonverbal communication occurs either singularly or in combination with verbal behaviors in the exchange and interpretation of messages within a given situation or context (Malandro, Barker, & Barker, 1989).

Approximately 50 to 90 percent of human communication is nonverbal. Consequently, messages are sent consciously and unconsciously through body movements, gestures, interpersonal space, and intonation.

Nonverbal communication behaviors have sometimes been classified into the following categories: **prosody, kinesics, proxemics,** and **paralanguage.**

1. **Prosody** refers to the melodic pattern of speech such as pitch, duration, loudness, and rhythm. Prosodic features carry meaning and may serve to confirm or contradict the spoken language. Stress and intonation may also be included (Thomas & Carmack, 1990). However, Owens (1988) adds that stress is a paralinguistic code that is employed to signal attitude or emotion. Problems in this area might include inappropriate responses and use of variations in pitch, duration, loudness, and rhythm.

2. **Kinesics** are the visual signals sent with the body to the receiver. Gestures, the eyes, and hands are often most commonly used to send visual body signals, either alone or in conjunction with a verbal message. These movements may transmit messages that either reinforce or contradict the spoken message. Problems can occur if the visual signals are misinterpreted by the receiver of the message or if the message sent by the visual signals are incongruent to the verbal message.

3. **Proxemics** is the distance of interpersonal and social space. Four categories of individual and social space have been identified by Goffman and Hall and reported by Stewart (1992) and Pritchett (1993):

- intimate
- personal
- social
- public

The amount of space people maintain between themselves and others generally provides information about relationships. Intimate space extends from actual physical contact outward, from six to eighteen inches. This space is usually reserved for those close to us. Personal space continues from eighteen inches outward to four feet; this is usually reserved for personal and business acquaintances. Social space encompasses distances from four to twelve feet from the body, during informal and formal social contacts. Public space includes everything from twelve feet and beyond.

In the classroom setting, effective proximity is defined as within about three feet of the student (Etscheidt, Stainback, & Stainback, 1984). Typically, people tend to move closer to others with the comfort of the relationship. By adjusting the distance, teachers and students suggest desired levels of involvement and convey messages about their level of interpersonal communication, i.e., intimate, aloof, intrusive, or neutral (Banbury & Hebert, 1992). Problems in this area can again occur with inappropriate actions or misinterpreted meanings within the area of proxemics.

4. Paralanguage is the production of sounds that are vocal, but nonverbal. Features of speech related to paralanguage include sounds that are produced in the vocal tract, but the sounds are not articulated speech sounds or words. According to Nicolosi, Harryman, and Krescheck (1989), paralanguage refers to features that are not part of the formal language system, but that are important to the comprehension and expression of that system, and includes body postures, facial expressions, hand gestures, stress, intonations, volume, and phrasing. Paralanguage may also express emotions. Active emotions, such as fear and anger, tend to be expressed by a fast rate of speech, loud volume, and high pitch. Passive emotions, such as sadness, are generally communicated by a slower rate of speech, lower volume and pitch, and a more resonant quality (Pritchett, 1993). Examples of paralanguage may also include yawning, grunting, laughing, or crying. Problems in this area can again occur with misinterpreted meanings within the area of paralanguage.

All four of these components can be culturally specific. For example, in the United States, nodding of the head generally indicates understanding or an affirmative answer, while in the Middle East this might signal an answer of "no" (Arthur, 1995). Differences in interpretations occur not only among cultures but also as a result of individualization and socialization processes. An understanding of these nonverbal communication techniques as they vary across different cultures and languages will assist the teacher in gaining much needed insight while providing instruction and interventions.

Owens (1994) adds that speech and language are but a part of communication. Other aspects of communication may serve to enhance or even eclipse the linguistic code. These aspects, as described by Owens (1988; 1994) are: paralinguistic, nonlinguistic, and metalinguistic:

- *paralinguistic mechanisms* change the form and meaning of a sentence by acting across individual sounds or words of a sentence, such as intonation (changes in pitch that signal the mood of an utterance), stress (employed for emphasis), rate of delivery (changes in speed that vary with the speaker's excitement, etc.), and pause or hesitation (breaks that can be used to emphasize a portion of the message or to replace the message);
- *nonlinguistic cues* include gestures, body posture, facial expression, eye contact, head and body movement, and physical distance or proxemics. Owens reminds us that the effectiveness of these cues may vary with users and between users;
- *metalinguistic cues* signal the status of communication based on our intuitions about the acceptability of utterances, including the ability to talk about language, analyze it, separate it from its context, and judge it. Owens further adds that these skills are used to judge the correctness or appropriateness of the language that we produce and receive.

Activities

- The next time you are at a public place (airport, mall, restaurant, elevator, etc.), specifically notice the distance (proxemics) between and among people. What conclusions can you draw from observations only?
- Within groups of four or five, one speaker will share a favorite story from the summer. While speaking, vary the pitch and loudness of the voice (prosody). What is the impact on the audience?
- Variation: When with your family or on a date, complete the same activity without sharing your intention. What are the reactions? Why do you think that this has happened?
- Within groups of four or five, discuss any type of disabilities in which voice, pitch, loudness, and rhythm may be a consistent problem. Describe some short- and long-term effects of this on both the speaker and the listener.

Language

Language is defined by the American Speech-Language-Hearing Association (ASHA) as a "complex and dynamic system of conventional symbols that is used in various modes for thought and communication" (ASHA, 1982). It is also viewed as a socially shared code or conventional system that is rule-governed, with specific conventions that are learned, a code in which specific symbols stand for something else (Owens, 1988; Hulit & Howard, 1993; Reed, 1994). The development of language is often heralded as the hallmark accomplishment of humans.

Language is unique to humans because only human beings can communicate their language by reading, writing, speaking, and listening. Language in humans is clearly dependent on their having a society (context) in which to learn it, other humans to speak to, and the intelligence to make it possible. Humans will acquire the language of those around them if they grow up around people who speak with them (Locke, 1990).

Children learn what language is by learning what language can do. This perspective on language acquisition that brings social aspects of the learning into prominence is called the "interactionist" view (Genishi & Dyson, 1984). Although prominent linguists maintained that every child is born with the universals of language "wired in" (Chomsky, 1964), the role of the environment is variously seen as shaping language learning through the reinforcement of selected responses, as prompting the child's language acquisition device, or as providing information from which the child can create and discard language rules. An environment that contains few reinforcers and few objects of interest to meet basic human needs is not a functional environment for learning or teaching language.

The development of language is a complex process. Young children normally progress through several stages in developing language; however, all children normally exhibit considerable variability in their stages of development. These differences may be due to general health, heredity, and environmental influences. Chapter 3, Early Communication Development, will comprehensively describe the developmental stages of language.

Over 6,000 different languages are spoken in the world (McLaughlin, 1998). Among these languages there exists a set of particular symbols and rules, a linguistic code, that users agree on to exchange information (Chomsky, 1969). Language is a formalized method of communication, and is comprised of systems of complex rules that govern components of language. These components, as described by Bloom & Lahey (1978), are: **form** (phonology, morphology, and syntax), **content** (semantics), and **use** (pragmatics).

A **language disorder** is defined by the American Speech-Language-Hearing Association as "the impairment or deviant development of comprehension and/or use of spoken, written and/or other symbol system" (ASHA, 1982, p. 949). The disorder may involve form, content, or use in any combination.

Components of Verbal Communication

Students with special needs have a higher prevalence of problems in language than other students. Five basic components of oral language are generally recognized: **phonology, morphology, syntax, semantics,** and **pragmatics.**

1. Phonology is the system of rules that governs sounds and their combination. Each language has specific sounds, or **phonemes,** that are characteristic of that language (Bernstein, 1984).

All the sounds used in human language, however diverse they may appear, can be described in terms of a limited set of sound vibrations relating to such factors as vibration of the vocal cords, air passage, shape of facial structures, and where the sounds are produced in the mouth. A phoneme is the smallest unit of sound in a word that makes a difference in its meaning. Forty-five sound elements (phonemes) create the phonological system of English (Heward, 2000). Although many language systems have common sounds, languages vary in the ways in which these sounds are produced and/or combined. Another important point here is that the sound system and written system are two different expressive systems, each with its own structure and conventions and uses. Phonological awareness involves an understanding that words can be divided into segments of sound smaller than a syllable, as well as knowledge, or awareness, of the identity of individual phonemes themselves. Therefore, phonological awareness is the ability to notice, think about, or manipulate the individual sounds in words (Torgesen, 1997). Often, the systems are confused with early speakers and writers. Examples of phonemes include /b/, /t/, /m/, and /d/. Problems of phonology might include the inability to produce phonemes and inadequate articulation sounds.

2. **Morphology** is the system of rules for combining sounds into meaningful units, such as words, suffixes, and prefixes. Simply stated, **morphemes** are the smallest linguistic units with meaning and form a bridge between phonology and syntax.

There are two basic types of morphemes: free and bound. **Free morphemes** can stand alone in a sentence, be used independently, and designate meaning. For example, all base words and root words are free morphemes because they cannot be broken down into smaller units, but convey meaning. Conversely, a **bound morpheme** is a grammatical marker that cannot function independently, so must be attached to free morphemes or to other bound morphemes. Examples generally include grammatical tags or markers that are derivational such as /-er/ or /-est/. Although bound morphemes convey no meaning independently, they provide grammatical information when added to free morphemes. For example, /-er/ and /-est/ signal comparisons, e.g., *short, shorter, shortest* and *fast, faster, fastest.*

Morphemes can be combined to form quite complex morphemes. Each combination, however, is bound by grammatical rules for meaning.

3. **Syntax.** The third component of form is **syntax.** Syntax refers to the arrangement of words combined by following the combinatory rule and patterns of the specific language to form meaningful sentences. For example, the English language relies heavily on the order of words to determine their meaning (Oyer, Hall, & Haas 1994; McLaughlin, 1998). The commonly held definition of a sentence is "a group of words that expresses a complete thought." Given that, a sentence involves relational meanings, as the various morphemes are connected to form the complete thought. A deep knowledge, understanding, and expert use of language

structure is very important when considering the syntax of a language. Problems of syntax might include sentence length, incompleteness, inability to organize verbal information, poor rote memory, and difficulty in understanding the relationship of word order to meaning.

4. **Semantics.** The content of language is referred to as the **semantics** of the language. Semantics refers to the ability to distinguish word meaning, including multiple meanings and subtle nuances, and to understand the language. Moreover, it is the meanings attached to words and word relationships (Mercer & Mercer, 1989).

Semanticists, specialists who study word meaning, view meaning as the essence of language and communication. Semantic knowledge is quite complex and constantly changing as knowledge of shades of meaning consistently add to the complexity of word meanings. It is in the semantic domain that language growth and development are most vigorous during the elementary school years.

Children who experience difficulties with this language component might have difficulty comprehending and expressing oral instructions, formulating sentences, differentiating between subtle differences in word meanings, and/or using expressive vocabulary. Other problems include experiencing difficulty in planning what to say, sequencing in a logical manner, and using grammatically correct sentences.

5. **Pragmatics.** The actual use of language within a social context is referred to as **pragmatics.** Moreover, it is the awareness of socially appropriate behaviors in communication interactions. Given that language is acquired and develops within a social context, pragmatics describe the physical and social context beyond the meaning of the words spoken (Hedge, 1995). Pragmatics include both the implicit and explicit social rules and conventions for communication, e.g., taking turns in a conversation, formality of language given the particular audience, and so on. Children who evidence problems with pragmatics may experience difficulty in interacting with peers, either verbally or socially.

Speech

Speech is the actual verbal process within communication. The production of sounds requires the coordination of oral neuromuscular movements to physically produce sound waves, the physical transmission of sound and meaning. The major components of speech are **articulation,** the production of sounds; **voice,** the vibration of the vocal cords; and, **fluency** or **rhythm,** the smoothness or flow of speech. A **speech disorder** is an impairment observed in the transmission and use of the oral symbol system that can be manifested as an **articulation disorder,** a **voice disorder,** or a **fluency disorder.**

Articulation

The production of the sound system of a language refers to articulation of speech sounds and speech patterns. **Distinctive features,** as the name implies, are used to describe and classify each speech sound in terms of the source of the sound in the vocal tract and the shape of the vocal tract during its production. If the source of the speech sound is a vocal cord vibration, it is called a "voiced" sound. Voiced sounds can be hummed or sung, at least for a fraction of a section, whereas "unvoiced" sounds cannot. An articulation disorder is the abnormal production of these speech sounds. There are four forms of misarticulations: errors of omission (*ta'* for *take);* errors of substitution (*yike* for *like);* errors of distortion (*zink* for *sink*) (in this case, there is noise added to the production of the *s* sound, yet not enough to be recorded as a substitution); and errors of addition (*boata* for *boat*).

Voice

Given all of the components of speech, language, and communication, voice is the closest measure of one's identity. Oftentimes, voice imparts identity, emotion, and personality. While voice is so important, it is often difficult to describe. The incidence of children with voice disorders may vary from as low as less than 1 percent to as high as 23 percent (Deal, McClain, & Sudderth, 1976.) Incidence may vary according to how data were gathered and evaluated, criteria used, and grade levels surveyed (Moore, 1986).

Disorders in the area of voice include disorders of pitch, loudness, and quality, or a combination of these factors. A speaker's pitch may be too high or too low for that particular person. Loudness, like pitch, may be a judgment of the listener. Poor vocal quality can be described as breathy, nasal, monotone, rough, harsh, strident, and grating. Problems with voice may be due to the physiological functioning of the vocal mechanism, ranging from situational causes of vocal misuse from screaming and yelling to much more serious causes such as vocal nodules, polyps, or cancer of the larynx.

Fluency

Fluent speech is relatively effortless, not punctuated with many irregularities, pauses, or discontinuities, and moves forward quite rhythmically and easily. Repeated interruptions, hesitations, and stops to the flow of speech may characterize fluency disorders. (Perkins, 1971; Van Riper, 1982; Bloodstein, 1987; and Shames & Rubin, 1986). Two of the most common types of fluency problems are stuttering and cluttering. The primary symptoms of **stuttering** are abnormally high frequency and long duration of sound, syllable, and word repetitions, as well as long durations for sound productions and pauses. While stuttering generally refers to an interruption in the rhythm and fluency of speech, **cluttering** refers to speech that is overly rapid, disorganized, and occasionally filled with unnecessary words and unrelated insertions.

Reflection

- Name the various components of communication, language, and speech. Develop various graphic organizers and mnemonics to assist your learning.
- Discuss which components of communication would be of greatest concern. What would you do as a classroom teacher with children that exhibit some of these concerns?

Changing Roles for Teachers

Federal Legislation

One of the first public school programs established to remediate speech problems began in Chicago in 1910, with several of the larger, urban school districts following within the next decade (Moore & Kester, 1953). Programs continued to expand, especially through the 1950s and 1960s. With the passage of two specific federal laws, services for all children with disabilities were guaranteed. Public Law 94-142, the Education for All Handicapped Children Act of 1975, mandated that all children with disabilities between the ages of five and eighteen were to receive free and appropriate education. Prior to the enactment of PL 94-142, it is estimated that over one million children were not receiving an education. Several years later, Public Law 99-457, the Education of the Handicapped Amendments of 1986, extended the right to free and appropriate public education to include children between the ages of three to kindergarten. Another provision of this law was the establishment of a state grant program for infants and toddlers up to the age of two years. Infants and toddlers who are defined by the state as developmentally delayed are eligible for services that include an individualized family service plan (IFSP) and a multidisciplinary assessment.

In 1990, and most recently in 1997, the original legislation of 1975 was reauthorized and renamed the Individuals with Disabilities Education Act (IDEA). This legislation is important for all students with disabilities. Services within the least restrictive environment are guaranteed for each child with a disability based on an individualized education plan (IEP). Teachers, parents, speech-language pathologists, health specialists, administrators, students, and others as appropriate, develop the individualized plan for students based on the specific educational needs of the students. Due to the critical importance of the individual education plan for each student receiving services, the reader is encouraged to seek much more information on both the procedures and policies governing this important process. (Readers are referred to introductory texts in special education for further information, e.g., Turnbull, Turnbull, Shank, & Leal, 1999; Hallahan & Kauffman, 1997; Heward, 2000; Hardman, Drew, & Egan, 1999.)

Communication disorders are one of the most prevalent disabling conditions among students in the United States today. Every school-aged child who is identified as having a communicative disorder (speech, language, or hearing) that adversely affects his or her educational achievement falls under the jurisdiction of IDEA. Once the appropriate identification and assessment procedures have been completed, an IEP must be designed and appropriate services implemented.

Evolving Roles for Teachers

In 1990–1991, 21 percent of the students up to the age of twenty-one with disabilities, who were being served under federal law, had speech or language impairments (U.S. Bureau of Census, 1993). Further, the *Sixteenth Annual Report to Congress* on the implementation of IDEA said that, next to learning disabilities, speech or language impairments were the most frequent disability receiving special services during the 1991–1992 school year (U.S. Department of Education, 1994).

Many children with communication disorders are not receiving an adequate amount of services from speech-language pathologists and audiologists (Casby, 1989). Thus, there is an even greater need for further involvement by special and general education teachers in helping students to communicate effectively (Hallahan & Kauffman, 1997).

Because of the legislation previously described, working as a team member in the schools to ensure that children with disabilities obtain an appropriate education will be of paramount concern to regular and special educators and speech-language pathologists. It is the regular and special educators who will be in an excellent position to identify language-related problems and to request assistance from the appropriately trained professional in that discipline. The Individualized Education Plan (IEP) further emphasizes the importance of collaboration. Team members may include a speech-language pathologist, a special education teacher, and a regular education teacher, a nurse, and a physical therapist, among many others.

Communication disorders have many causes and reveal themselves in many different ways. Therefore, there is no one profession that can provide all the remediation services needed for individuals with communication disorders (Boone & Plante, 1997). As an integral member of this interactive team, it is imperative that individual differences in roles and perspectives be realized, for these can be viewed as assets if they are respected by all team members and used appropriately by the team leader (Morsink, Thomas, & Correa, 1991). Further, as more school districts move toward inclusion, both regular and special education teachers will be expected to have expertise in a broad array of disabilities.

The American Speech-Language-Hearing Association (ASHA) and the Council for Exceptional Children (CEC) have both played key roles in furthering the evolving roles for teachers. ASHA, the national governing organization of speech-language pathologists and audiologists, and CEC, the professional organization of special education, both have mission statements emphasizing the need for collaboration across disciplines. Both organizations will be further discussed in a subsequent chapter.

Activities

- Follow a speech-language pathologist or an audiologist. Try to identify the types of problems exhibited by the students that you observed.
- Observe a group of youngsters in a play setting. Identify the categories of language that you observe.
- Attend an IEP or an IFSP staffing. Identify the team members present and their roles and responsibilities.
- With a peer, design an activity that will assist you in understanding the various components of verbal and nonverbal communication.

Overview

The American Speech-Language-Hearing Association (ASHA) distinguishes between disorders of communication and variations in communication that are not disorders and defines them (ASHA, 1982) (Figure 1.2). Many of these topics will be covered in subsequent chapters, including voice, articulation, fluency, and language disorders. Other topics to be covered throughout the text include: the culturally and linguistically diverse exceptional student, the student with a hearing disorder, augmentative/assistive technology, special populations, and children who exhibit mild impairments of learning, those with intellectual deficits, and individuals with emotional problems.

Throughout this text, it is hoped that the reader will be constantly reminded that the remediation of communication problems in children does not lie with any single profession (Hallahan & Kauffman, 1997; Matthews & Frattali, 1994). Figure 1.3 shows the range of disciplines and professionals concerned with communication disorders. While the disciplines of speech-language pathology and audiology have communication disorders as their central concern (Matthews & Frattali, 1994), it is the classroom teacher and the special education teacher who may identify the possible communication problem and intervene as necessary to refer the student to the appropriate hearing or speech professional.

The following chapters will elaborate and detail the preliminary discussions and definitions presented here. It is hoped that, as readers continue to study and read these chapters, the terms and definitions outlined in this chapter will serve as a framework. It is our desire to provide information and strategies that the classroom teacher might use to become a more informed and contributing member of the collaborative team.

FIGURE 1.2   *Definitions of the American Speech-Language-Hearing Association*

Communicative Disorders	*Communicative Variations*
A. A SPEECH DISORDER is an impairment of voice, articulation of speech sounds, and/or fluency. These impairments are observed in the transmission and use of the oral symbol system.	A. COMMUNICATIVE DIFFERENCE/DIALECT is a variation of a symbol system used by a group of individuals that reflects and is determined by shared regional, social, or cultural/ethnic factors. Variations or alterations in the use of a symbol system may be indicative of primary language inferences. A regional, social, or cultural/ethnic variation of a symbol system should not be considered a disorder of speech or language.

A. A SPEECH DISORDER is an impairment of voice, articulation of speech sounds, and/or fluency. These impairments are observed in the transmission and use of the oral symbol system.

  1. A VOICE DISORDER is defined as the absence or abnormal production of voice quality, pitch, loudness, resonance, and/or duration.

  2. An ARTICULATION DISORDER is defined as the abnormal production of speech sounds.

  3. A FLUENCY DISORDER is defined as the abnormal flow of verbal expression, characterized by impaired rate and rhythm which may be accompanied by struggle behavior.

B. A LANGUAGE DISORDER is the impairment or deviant development of comprehension and/or use of a spoken, written and/or symbol system. The disorder may involve (1) the form of language (phonologic, morphologic, and syntactic systems), (2) the content of language (semantic system), and/or (3) the function of language in communication (pragmatic system) in any combination.

  1. Form of Language

    a. PHONOLOGY is the sound system of a language and the linguistic rules that govern the sound combinations.

    b. MORPHOLOGY is the linguistic rule system that governs the structure of words and the construction of word forms from the basic elements of meaning.

    c. SYNTAX is the linguistic rule governing the order and combination of words to form sentences, and the relationships among the elements within a sentence.

  2. Content of Language

    a. SEMANTICS is the psycholinguistic system that patterns the content of an utterance—the intent and meanings of words and sentences.

  3. Function of Language

    a. PRAGMATICS is the sociolinguistic system that patterns the use of language in communication which may be expressed motorically, vocally, or verbally.

A. COMMUNICATIVE DIFFERENCE/DIALECT is a variation of a symbol system used by a group of individuals that reflects and is determined by shared regional, social, or cultural/ethnic factors. Variations or alterations in the use of a symbol system may be indicative of primary language inferences. A regional, social, or cultural/ethnic variation of a symbol system should not be considered a disorder of speech or language.

B. AUGMENTATIVE COMMUNICATION is a system used to supplement the communicative skills of individuals for whom speech is temporarily or permanently inadequate to meet communicative needs. Both prosthetic devices and/or nonprosthetic techniques may be designed for individual use as an augmentative communication system.

Source: American Speech-Language-Hearing Association, Definitions: Communicative disorders and variations, ASHA, 24 (1982), 949–950.

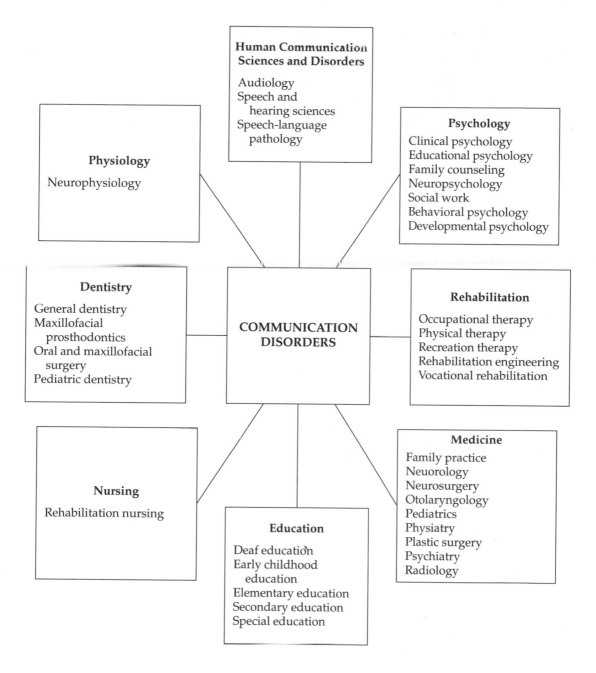

FIGURE 1.3 *Disciplines and Professions Related to Human Communication Disorders*

Source: Matthews, L., & Frattali, C. Disciplines and professions related to human communication disorders. In G. H. Shames, E. H. Wiig, & W. A. Secord (Eds.), *Human communication disorders: An introduction* (4th ed). Copyright © 1994 by Allyn & Bacon.

> *Reflection*
>
> **To enhance your understanding of the introductory information regarding speech and language development and disorders, reflect on and complete the following activity: Begin a portfolio of all the readings, reflections, and assignments that will be discussed in this class relative to speech, language, and communication.**

Summary

This introductory chapter provides the reader with a basic understanding of the terms and concepts in the areas of language and speech and associated communicative problems. It is hoped that this knowledge will enhance your understanding of communication problems exhibited by some of the youngsters in your classroom. The next chapters will all build on your understanding of these important concepts that you have mastered. Good luck and good learning.

This chapter has presented a preview and overview of communication and language. Communication does not occur in isolation. There must, at least, be a sender, a message, and a receiver. We've also learned that communication, language, and speech are highly complex skills that develop as a result of many supportive processes. All three terms—communication, language, and speech—describe different, related, and overlapping aspects of human behavior. Defining these terms should serve you well in understanding the processes involved.

Subsequent chapters will elaborate and detail the preliminary discussions and definitions presented here. It is suggested that, as you study the chapters, you use this chapter to review terms and concepts.

References and Suggested Readings

American Speech-Language-Hearing Association. (1982, November). Definitions: Communicative disorders and variations. *ASHA, 24,* 949–950.

Arthur, D. (1995, June). The importance of body language. *HR Focus, 72* (6), 22–26.

Banbury, M., & Hebert, C. (1992). Do you see what I mean? Body language in classroom interactions. *TEACHING Exceptional Children, 24*(4), 194–198.

Bernstein, R. (1984). Cues to post-vocalic voicing in mother-child speech. *Journal of Phonetics, 12,* 285–289.

Bloodstein, O. (1987). *A handbook on stuttering* (4th ed.). Chicago: National Easter Seals Society.

Bloom, L., & Lahey, M. (1978). *Language development and language disorders.* New York: John Wiley & Sons.

Boone, D. R., & Plante, E. (1997). *Human communication and its disorders* (2nd ed.). Boston: Allyn & Bacon.

Casby, M. W. (1989). National data concerning communication disorders and special education. *Language, Speech, and Hearing Services in the Schools, 20,* 22–30.

Chomsky, C. (1969). *The acquisition of syntax in children from 5 to 10.* Cambridge, MA: MIT Press.

Chomsky, N. (1964). Current issues in linguistic theory. In J. Fodor & J. Katz (Eds.), *The structure of language* (pp. 55–118). Englewood Cliffs, NJ: Prentice-Hall.

Committee on Language, American Speech-Language-Hearing Association. (1983, June). *ASHA, 25,* 44.

Deal, R. E., McClain, B., & Sudderth, J. F. (1976). Identification, evaluation, therapy, and follow-up for children with vocal nodules in a public school setting. *Journal of Speech and Hearing Disorders, 41,* 390–397.

Etscheidt, S., Stainback, S., & Stainback, W. (1984). The effectiveness of teacher proximity as an initial technique of helping students control their behavior. *Pointer, 28*(4), 33–35.

Genishi, C., & Dyson, A. H. (1984). *Language assessment in the early years.* Norwood, NJ: Ablex.

Gleason, J. B. (1993). *The development of language.* New York: Macmillan.

Hallahan, D. P., & Kaufman, J. M. (1997). *Exceptional learners: An introduction to special education.* Boston: Allyn & Bacon.

Hardman, M., Drew, C., & Egan, M. (1999). *Human exceptionality* (6th ed.). Boston: Allyn & Bacon.

Hedge, M. N. (1995). *Introduction to communicative disorders* (2nd ed.). Austin, TX: PRO-ED.

Heward, W. L. (2000). *Exceptional children: An introduction to special education* (6th ed.). Upper Saddle River, NJ: Merrill/Prentice-Hall.

Hulit, L. M., & Howard, M. R. (1993). *Born to talk: An introduction to speech and language development.* New York: Macmillan.

Hymes, D. (1974). *Foundations of sociolinguistics: An ethnographic approach.* Philadelphia: University of Pennsylvania Press.

Kirk, S., Gallagher, J., & Anastasiow, N. (2000). *Educating exceptional children* (9th ed.). Boston: Houghton Mifflin.

Lindfors, J. W. (1987). *Children's language and learning* (2nd ed.). Englewood Cliffs, NJ: Prentice-Hall.

Locke, J. (1990). Structure and stimulation is the ontogeny of spoken language. *Developmental Psychology, 23* (7), 621–644.

Malandro, L. A., Barker, L., & Barker, D. (1989). *Nonverbal communication.* New York: Random House.

Mastropieri, M. A., & Scruggs, T. E. (2000). *The inclusive classroom: Strategies for effective instruction.* Upper Saddle River, NJ: Merrill/Prentice-Hall.

Matthews, L., & Frattali, C. (1994). The professions of speech-language pathology and audiology. In G. H. Shames, E. H. Wiig, & W. A. Secord (Eds.), *Human communication disorders: An introduction* (4th ed., pp. 2–33). Boston: Allyn & Bacon.

McColgin, L. S. (1988). *The speech and language glossary.* Denver, CO: Communication Skill Builders.

McLaughlin, S. (1998). *Introduction to language development.* San Diego, CA: Singular Publishing Group.

Mercer, C., & Mercer, A. (1989). *Teaching students with learning problems* (5th ed.). Englewood Cliffs, NJ: Prentice-Hall.

Moore, G. (1986). Voice disorders. In G. H. Shames & E. H. Wiig (Eds.), *Human communication disorders* (2nd ed, pp. 183–241). Boston: Allyn & Bacon

Moore, G. P., & Kester, D. (1953). Historical notes on speech correction in the preassociation era. *Journal of Speech and Hearing Disorders, 10,* 48–53.

Morsink, C., Thomas, C., & Correa, V. (1991). *Interactive teaming: Consultation and collaboration in special programs.* New York: Merrill.

Nicolosi, L., Harryman, E., & Krescheck, J. (1989). *Terminology of communication disorders: Speech-language hearing* (3rd ed.). Baltimore, MD: Williams & Wilkins.

Owens, R. (1988). *Language development: An introduction* (2nd ed.). Columbus, OH: Merrill.

Owens, R. (1994). Development of communication, language, and speech. In G. H. Shames, E. H. Wiig, & W. A. Secord (Eds.), *Human communication disorders: An introduction* (4th ed., pp. 36–82). New York: Merrill/Macmillan.

Owens, Jr., R. E. (1999). *Language disorders: A functional approach to assessment and intervention* (3rd ed.). Boston: Allyn & Bacon.

Oyer, H., Hall, B., & Haas, W. (1994). *Speech, language, and hearing disorders: A guide for the teacher.* Boston: Allyn & Bacon.

Perkins, W. H. (1971). *Speech pathology: An applied behavior science.* St Louis, MO: Mosby.

Pritchett, G. L. (1993, July). Interpersonal communication. *FBI Law Enforcement Bulletin, 62*(7), 22–26.

Reed, V. A. (1994). *An introduction to children with language disorders* (2nd ed.). New York: Macmillan/Merrill.

Shames, G. H., & Rubin, H. (Eds.). (1986). *Stuttering then and now.* Columbus, OH: Charles E. Merrill.

Stewart, S. (1992, December) Too close for comfort? *Current Health 2, 19*(4), 4–6.

Thomas, P., & Carmack, F. (1990). *Speech and language: Detecting and correcting special needs.* Boston: Allyn & Bacon.

Torgesen, J. (1997). Phonological awareness. Paper presented to Florida State Department of Education.

Turnbull, A., Turnbull, R., Shank, M., & Leal, D. (1999). *Exceptional lives: Special education in today's schools* (2nd ed.). Upper Saddle River, NJ: Merrill/Prentice-Hall.

U.S. Bureau of Census. (1993). Current populations reports (Series P-60, No. 181). Washington, DC: U.S. Department of Education, Office of Educational Research and Improvement, National Center for Educational Statistics.

U.S. Department of Education, Office of Special Education Programs. (1994). *Sixteenth Annual Report to Congress on the Implementation of the Individuals with Disabilities Education Act.* Washington, DC: Author.

Van Riper, C. (1982). *The nature of stuttering* (2nd ed.). Englewood Cliffs, NJ: Prentice-Hall.

Van Riper, C., & Erickson, R. L. (1996). *Speech correction: An introduction to speech pathology and audiology* (9th ed.). Boston: Allyn & Bacon.

2

The Speech Process:
How It Works

Martha S. Lue

Chapter Objectives _____

On completion of this chapter, the reader will be able to:

- Explain the speech process;
- Understand the systems of the body involved in that process; and
- Describe how these systems work together to produce speech sounds.

- Ms. Jones decided to take her daughter's new tape player to her pre-school class. For many of the students in Ms. Jones's preschool class, this was their first experience with a tape recorder. The tape recorder is very attractive, made with primary colors, with a microphone attached to it. The children all became excited when they saw it. They all wanted to talk first. The goal was for all of them to be able to hear their voice. Some students would yell into it and make funny noises, while others would giggle a lot. Finally all took turns talking into the microphone. Some of the youngsters remained reluctant to talk, but while they were playing at the sand table, the teacher turned the tape player on without their knowing it. When they finally had an opportunity to listen to the tape, they would say things like, "Is that me?" or "That's me." As a matter of fact, they would get very excited when they heard their voice. All in all, this became a fun day at preschool.

- Sara, a three-year-old, is a student at the Early Intervention Center. She was born with five holes in her heart, commonly referred to as heart murmurs. She has had four surgeries to close the holes, but still has two holes present. She is on medications for seizures, which are believed to have been caused by the heart murmurs. The medications have many side effects, which have slowed her development. The condition also caused her to be sick more often and longer than usual. This condition is genetic. Her older brother has Down syndrome. Even though it is not known if Sara has other problems, this condition has caused her to have learning and speech problems as well as some physical disabilities. She was just one year old when she began to crawl and was two when she began to walk. She is below the expected weight for children of her age. Every other day, she goes to a speech therapist, and other days she goes to a physical therapist to help her use her arms and legs.

- Julian is one of a set of twins. Three weeks after he and his twin were born, it was discovered that he had Down syndrome. After going through periods of crying and sadness, the family accepted the diagnosis and began to adjust to having a child with special needs in the family. His twin sister has developed normally with no identified physical or intellectual problems. His family feels that he is mildly mentally handicapped with minimal physical problems, including ear infections, sinusitis, and a compromised immune system. He started walking when he was two-and-a-half years of age. His expressive vocabulary, even at the age of eight years, is very small and limited. His receptive vocabulary is far greater than his expressive vocabulary. His best words are *hi* and *bye*. He is also learning sign language.

  Julian currently attends a mainstreamed class for library, music, art, lunch, gym, and recess. The rest of the day he spends either in his special education classroom or with the occupational, physical, or speech therapists. He engages in many extracurricular activities, where he has taken swimming lessons and played T-ball on a team with children with disabilities. The family has been involved in a support group for families of children with Down syndrome, and they are preparing for the day that he will become an independent adult.

- Martin, nine years old, suffered a closed-head injury and, as a result, has had severe deficits in both spoken and written language. His spoken language is extremely slow and labored. He pauses between each syllable in a word and has trouble articulating many sounds. Additionally, he exhibits oral motor problems and drools frequently. The salivation problem also slows his speech as he has to pause often to swallow or wipe his mouth.

Another concern is Martin's written output. Because of the physical effects of his injury, he has lost almost all fine motor control. He also has a severe tremor that extremely limits his control. He is therefore unable to write. The occupational therapist and other professionals have been working for weeks on an alternate means of written communication that would be effective for this student. Due to his tremor, using a regular computer keyboard is out of the question. Even with a key guard, the keys were too small and his accuracy was extremely poor. Therefore, a flat keyboard is now being tried, where the area for each letter is larger than that of a regular keyboard. On top of this, there is a key guard, providing the student with a place to rest his hands to reduce the effect of his tremors. In addition, he must either hold his wrist or wear a small weight around his wrist to control the shaking. Even with these accommodations, Martin has a great deal of trouble typing letters accurately.

Of all the acts a human being does, none seems quite as complex as the act of speaking and the speech process itself. The speech process represents and reflects what makes human beings different from other animals in our ability to communicate.

Listening to one's voice, even at an early age, as demonstrated by the youngsters in *Ms. Jones*'s preschool class, can be an exciting and exhilarating experience. The voice of a child making its first sounds is both welcomed and reassuring to new parents. The speech act is very complex and is nothing short of a miracle. In fact, the process is more complicated and more versatile than any instrument found in a symphony orchestra (Van Riper & Erickson, 1996). It involves multiple systems, all working together to bring forth verbal communication. But sometimes, as illustrated in the cases presented by *Sara, Julian,* and *Martin,* children do not learn to speak or may experience difficulty in learning to speak or in the act of speaking because of developmental, physiological, or acquired disabilities, although they can communicate in some limited fashion by using the neurophysical systems under their control. TV programs and movies are filled with the fateful moment when the coma victim manages to blink his eyes or squeeze a hand in response to a question directed her way.

As an educator, you will see children who speak normally and those for whom speech presents a challenge or who may not be able to speak at all. This chapter will analyze the speech process, discuss the systems of the body involved in that process, and describe how these systems and processes work together to produce speech sounds. Speech is the product of four separate but inextricably linked systems: respiration, phonation, resonance, and articulation (Figures 2.1 and 2.2).

Several texts provide detailed information on the anatomy and physiology of speech (Dickson & Maue-Dickson, 1988; Seikel, King, & Drumright, 1997; Shearer, 1979; Kahane, 1986; Schneiderman, 1984; Zemlin, 1994). It is our intent to present the systems and associated structures that contribute to speech production (respiration, phonation, resonance, and articulation) in terms that are meaningful to you

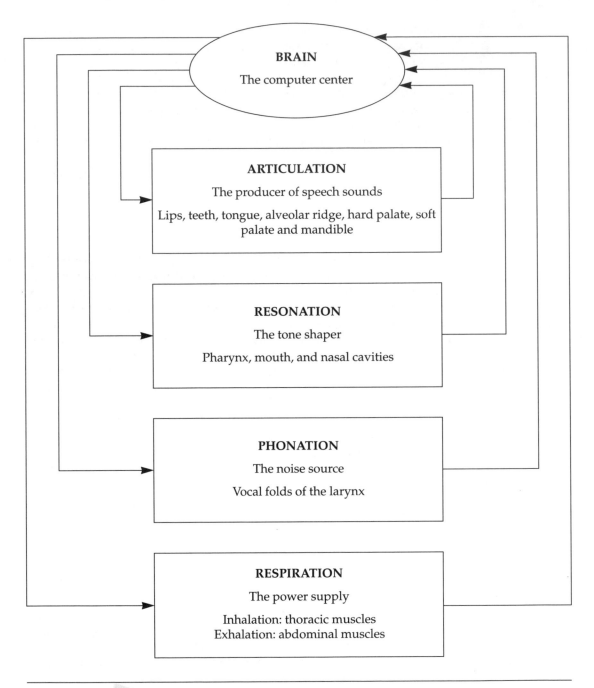

FIGURE 2.1 *The Processes of Speech*

Source: From L. M. Hulit and M. R. Howard, *Born to Talk.* Copyright © 1993 by Allyn & Bacon. All rights reserved. Reprinted by permission of Allyn & Bacon.

as an educator. Please be reminded that these systems do not function independently of one another during communication; to the contrary, they function almost simultaneously during the speech process.

In humans, one or the other of the systems associated with speech production may be underdeveloped or damaged, as in the cases of Sara, Julian, and Martin. Sometimes one of the other systems may be developed or trained to afford compensation with resulting communication occurring. Educators and speech-language pathologists are often the professionals who work with individuals to adapt through other systems. In Chapter 11, mechanical aides to assist individuals with disabilities will be discussed. We will begin this discussion with a brief examination of the central nervous system.

Reflection

- **Try to make it through one day, or at least half a day, without using your voice. What are some alternative methods you can find to communicate with others?**
- **As we learn more about technological advances in all aspects of our daily lives, what do you think is the possibility that missing parts of the speech mechanism can be genetically cloned or that cranial nerves will be transplanted from one individual to another?**

The Central Nervous System

The Central Nervous System (CNS) represents the command center. It is the major area for origination, planning, and transmitting both conscious thought and deliberate actions and autonomic involuntary messages. If the maturation of the central nervous system is delayed, the child may be slow to talk.

The CNS consists of the brain and spinal cord. The brain is divided into two halves or hemispheres. These hemispheres are connected by several structures that allow the communication of messages between the hemispheres and transmission of messages up and down the spinal cord. The area between the spinal cord and hemispheres is called the **brain stem.** The brain stem is the main life support control system of the body.

The largest part of the brain is called the **cerebrum.** The cerebrum is considered the most important structure of the central nervous system for speech, language, and hearing. Each lobe of the cerebrum is divided into four regions: frontal lobe, occipital lobe, parietal lobe, and temporal lobe. Functions of the lobes include:

Frontal lobe: Controls the voluntary muscles, especially those involving speech production. Broca's area, an important motor speech center, is found in the left frontal lobe.

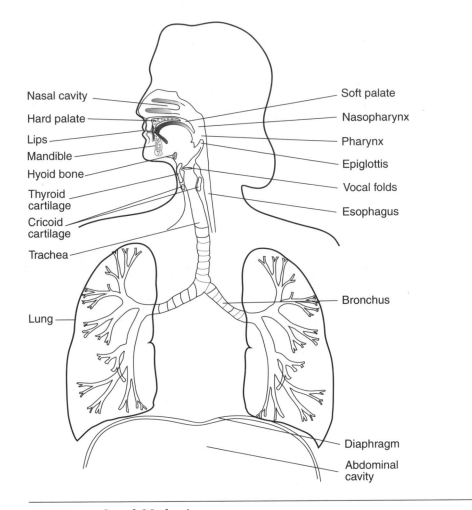

FIGURE 2.2 *Speech Mechanism*
Courtesy of John Albritton, M.D.

Occipital lobe: Located at the lower back portion of the head, above the cerebellum; primarily concerned with vision, including visual perception and recognition.

Parietal lobe: Concerned with pressure, pain, temperature, and muscular sensations; it may also be vital for overall sensorimotor functioning.

Temporal lobe: Contains the primary auditory context, which receives the sound stimuli from the auditory nerve (cranial nerve VIII). Toward the back of the brain stem is the **cerebellum,** which controls coordination for the smoothness of movements programmed by the hemispheres.

A fluid that protects and cushions them, called *cerebrospinal fluid*, surrounds the brain and spinal cord. An accumulation of cerebrospinal fluid can lead to a condition called *hydrocephalus*.

Geschwind (1979) observes that the human brain is distinguishable because of its ability to learn a variety of activities; the most complex activity is that of language. Disagreement, however, still persists on what effect, if any, the two hemispheres have on language (Munsell, Rauen, & Kinjo, 1988).

Reflection

- **Begin your own list of mnemonic devices that will assist you in remembering some complex information and terms, such as "CAT"—Cricoid, Arytenoid, Thyroid cartilages.**
- **Begin your list of affixes and suffixes that will aid you in unscrambling some difficult terms:** *a,* **absence of (***aphonia,* **"absence or loss of voice");** *gloss,* **"tongue" (***glossopharyngeal,* **the cranial nerve that innervates muscles of the tongue and pharynx).**

The Cranial Nerves

The brain serves as the origin or terminal for twelve pairs of nerves called cranial nerves, so called because they enter or exit the same structural space that is occupied by the brain, the skull (Hedge, 1995). Almost two-thirds of these nerves are devoted to the innervation of the larynx and upper airway articulators. Simply stated, seven of those pairs are important in speech or hearing: V (trigeminal), VII (facial), VIII (auditory), IX (glossopharyngeal), X (vagus), XI (spinal accessory), and XII (hypoglossal). Five pairs are not concerned with speech or hearing. Cranial nerve I (olfactory) is concerned with smell. Cranial nerves II (optic), III (oculomotor), IV (trochlear), and VI (abducens) are related to vision and the movement of the eyes. A complete listing of the nerves and their general function is found in Table 2.1.

Cranial nerves that bring sensory information to the brain from the body are called **sensory.** Those that send impulses to the muscles to produce movement are called **motor.** Some, which serve both functions, are called *mixed.* A brief discussion of those cranial nerves important for speech and hearing follows. Their numbers and names identify them.

Cranial Nerve V—Trigeminal (Mixed).   The largest of the cranial nerves, *tri* indicates that it has three branches:

Ophthalmic: Sensory fibers from the skin over the upper eyelid; upper part of the nasal cavity; anterior half of the scalp.

Maxillary: Receives sensory impulses from the mucosa of the nose, palate, upper teeth, upper lip, cheek, and lower eyelid.

TABLE 2.1   *The Cranial Nerves, Their Names, Functions, and Potential Roles in Speech Language.*

No.	Name	Function	Potential Role in Speech-Language
I	Olfactory	Sensory: Smell	Associating smells
II	Optic	Sensory: Vision	Associating physical features
III	Oculomotor	Motor: Eye movement	Searching/tracking movement
IV	Trochlear	Motor: Eye movement	Searching/tracking movement
V	Trigeminal	Sensory: Face Motor: Jaw	Moving jaw for feeding/speech
VI	Abducens	Motor: Eye movement	Searching/tracking movement
VII	Facial	Sensory: Tongue Motor: Jaw	Controlling jaw and tongue; associating tastes; facial expressions
VIII	Vestibular Acoustic	Sensory: Hearing	Associating sounds, including speech, sensations, and balance
IX	Glossopharyngeal	Sensory: Tongue	Controlling palate and pharynx for speech
X	Vagus	Sensory and Motor: Larynx	Controlling larynx for phonation; Lungs, heart, esophagus, stomach
XI	Spinal Accessory	Motor: Shoulder, larynx	Controlling shoulder for respiration; also larynx, and pharynx
XII	Hypoglossal	Motor: Tongue movements	Controlling tongue for articulation

Reprinted with permission by Singular Publishing Group, Inc. *Introduction to Language Development,* S. McLaughlin, Singular Publishing Group, San Diego, CA © 1998.

Mandibular: Carries motor fibers that supply the muscles of the mandible and the soft palate.

The trigeminal nerve is anesthetized in dental procedures. Injury to the nerve can cause paralysis of the muscles of mastication and loss of sensation of touch and temperature. If there is partial paralysis of the face, or faulty control of the mandible, that affects articulation.

Cranial Nerve VII Facial (Mixed).   This nerve has two branches:

> Motor: Muscles of facial expression, tear glands, and external ear.
>
> Sensory: Anterior two-thirds of tongue, soft palate, and adjacent pharynx. Injury to this nerve can produce paralysis of the facial muscles, as in the condition Bell's palsy. In Bell's palsy, there is a unilateral paralysis of the face that may be characterized by impaired hearing, disturbed speech, and distorted features (Nicolosi, Harryman, & Kresheck, 1978).

Cranial Nerve VIII: Auditory (Sensory).   This nerve is important for transmitting sound and balance sensation from the inner ear to the brain. Its two branches are:

> Cochlear: Conveys impulses associated with hearing.
> Vestibular: Conveys impulses associated with equilibrium.

Injury to the cochlear branch may cause "ringing" in the ears, known as *tinnitus.* Injury to the vestibular branch can cause vertigo (dizziness). Damage may arise, for example, from physical trauma to the skull or from tumor growth.

Cranial Nerve IX: Glossopharyngeal (Mixed).   Its major functions include innervating some pharyngeal muscles, and it serves general and taste sensations in the back part of the tongue and in the pharynx.

Cranial Nerve X: Vagus or Pneumogastric (Mixed).   Its functions include contributing to the motor control of the soft palate (velum), pharynx (throat), and larynx (voice box). This nerve is commonly referred to as the "vagus" because it wanders from the soft palate through many other parts of the body, including the trunk and the abdomen.

Cranial Nerve XI: Spinal Accessory (Motor).   Its function includes innervating large strap muscles of the head, neck, and shoulders, thus potentially influencing the position of the larynx and rib cage. It also supplies the muscles of the soft palate and the pharynx.

Cranial Nerve XII: Hypoglossal (Motor).   This nerve innervates muscles of the tongue. If there is difficulty with cranial nerve XII, the tongue deviates and may become atrophied. Many speech sounds may be slurred.

In discussing cranial nerves, it may be important to note that some people suffer from multiple cranial nerve palsies, such as in Guillain-Barre syndrome. This syndrome may begin with unilateral weakness or paralysis, most commonly beginning in the lower extremities. It attacks various nerves until the individual becomes completely debilitated.

Activity

Using the Internet, look for some of the latest research on the brain. Design a brief presentation of your findings for your classmates.

The Respiratory System

The respiratory system is our energy source for life in general and speech in particular. It ensures that oxygen is supplied to and waste carbon dioxide is removed from the body's cells. The respiratory system helps to maintain a constant environment that enables our body cells to function properly. Secondarily, it provides the power for phonation (Schneiderman, 1984).

While respiration covers the entire process of gaseous exchanges in the smallest cells of the body, breathing is that limited division of respiration in which air enters and leaves the lungs providing the medium for oxygen to be removed in the lungs to begin circulation to the cells ultimately for oxidation. The process of respiration requires the movement of air into and out of the lungs during inhalation and exhalation (Dickson & Maue-Dickson, 1988).

Breathing *in* is known as inspiration or inhalation. In the inhalation process, air enters the mouth and/or the nose. From these areas, the air passes into the pharynx, which links the nasal and oral cavities to the larynx and esophagus. The esophagus, a tube extending downward from the pharynx to the stomach, opens into the larynx. Approximately 50 percent of each breathing cycle is spent on inhalation, and about 50 percent on exhalation. Breathing for speech, however, is different. During speech, approximately 15 percent of the breathing cycle is devoted to inhalation and 85 percent to exhalation (Hulit & Howard, 1993). Breathing *out* is known as expiration or exhalation. Breathing, in the exhalation cycle, provides the energy for upward movement of the breath stream, which is then modified in a number of ways to form sound and speech. However, during conversational speech, the abdominal muscles are contracted for both expiration and inspiration. The breathing process, as a part of respiration, begins at the mouth and nose openings and terminates deep within the lungs.

Structurally, the respiratory system is divided into two areas, the upper and lower respiratory tracts. The larynx, pharynx, and oral and nasal cavities comprise the upper respiratory tract. The lower respiratory tract consists of the trachea, all segments of the bronchial tree, and the lungs. Associated functioning support structures are the rib cage, with its twelve pairs of ribs, the chest (thorax) and abdominal muscles, and the diaphragm, a muscle layer separating the thoracic and the abdominal cavities. The diaphragm and the chest walls create the vacuum, which controls the intake and outgo of air from the lungs.

Air flows in through the mouth and nose, down through the pharynx, on downward through the trachea, and bronchial tubes, finally reaching and inflating the lungs. Air is taken into the lungs as a normal part of the breathing cycle for about 2.5 seconds per breath and then expelled.

The first modification of the upward-moving breath stream takes place in the larynx, by vibration of the vocal folds, to add sound or "voice" whenever a voiced sound is required. This process of generating sound is called **phonation.**

The Phonation Mechanism

The Phonatory System

While phonation is produced by the vibration of the vocal folds in the larynx, the phonatory system involves the coordination of many muscles, organs, and structures in the abdomen, chest, throat, and head (Sataloff, 1992). Researchers suggest that "virtually the entire body influences the sound of the voice, either directly or indirectly" (Sataloff, 1992). This mechanism includes the sound-producing structures, the larynx and the vocal folds and the major cartilages of the larynx. A cartilage may be defined as a tissue that is considered softer and more flexible than bone.

The Larynx.　　The **larynx** (voice box) is the chief organ of phonation and represents the first stage of sound production and modification. It is located in the neck between the root of the tongue and the trachea (windpipe). It serves four biological functions (Zemlin, 1994):

Closing the airway to protect the lungs from food and liquids;

Impounding the air, thereby stabilizing the rib cage for more efficient muscle support in lifting;

Impounding the air for increasing internal abdominal pressure, as in bearing down; and

Holding the airway open to allow easy inhalation and exhalation.

The larynx also serves a social function—the production of voice for both verbal and nonverbal sounds for communication (Stevens, 1992; Sataloff, 1992). Located above the larynx is a U-shaped bone called the *hyoid.* It supports the larynx from above and serves a vital role in moving the larynx up during the act of swallowing. Above the larynx is yet another structure, called the **epiglottis.** Made of cartilage, this structure serves an important role when we swallow—it prevents food from entering the lungs.

From each side of the top of the larynx, paired folds of muscle tissue, lined by mucous membrane, appear as transverse folds that constitute the **vocal folds.** Phonation is produced primarily by these folds located on either side of the larynx. The folds are thicker in men than women and thicker in adults than in prepubescent children, thus accounting for the pitch differences found in these age and sex groups.

Glottis.   The **glottis** is the small opening between the vocal folds when the folds are adducted (closed). During normal breathing, the glottis is open. During full voice, the folds are closed, and the glottis disappears (Hulit & Howard, 1993).

Three major cartilages surround the larynx: thyroid, arytenoid, and cricoid cartilages.

Thyroid Cartilage.   The **thyroid cartilage,** the largest of the cartilages, is often called the "Adam's Apple." It forms an anterior wall for the larynx and protects its interior, and consists of two halves united at an angle, called the *laryngeal prominence.* The vocal folds are attached at their sides to the wall of the thyroid cartilage.

Arytenoid Cartilage.   At the back, each of the vocal folds is attached to a pyramid-shaped cartilage known as the arytenoid. The arytenoid can pivot or rotate, tilt backward, or slide backward and sideways. **Arytenoid cartilages** are paired cartilages.

Cricoid Cartilage.   A ring-shaped cartilage, the **cricoid cartilage,** lies directly below the thyroid cartilage and forms the foundation or base of the larynx.

The Resonation System

After passage through the vocal folds, the next stage of modification takes place in the pharynx, mouth, and nose or nasal cavities. This process is called resonating, and gives each person a unique voice quality. Whereas the chief organ of phonation is the larynx, the chief organ of resonance is the pharynx, or throat cavity. **Resonance** is "the process wherein certain frequencies in the laryngeal tones are reinforced or emphasized depending upon the size and shape of the speech resonators, including the pharynx, mouth and nasal cavities" (Hulit & Howard, 1993).

Other areas of resonance include the oral and nasal cavities. Nasal resonance occurs when sounds such as *m, n, ng* (as in *mother, nose,* and *sing*) are made. However, if there is too much nasal resonance in our speech, a condition known as **hypernasality** (*hyper* = "over") may be recognized. On the other hand, if too little resonance is present, **hyponasality** (*hypo* = "under") is diagnosed.

The Articulation System

The final modification of the breath stream is **articulation**—the molding, shaping, stopping, and releasing of voiced and nonvoiced sounds of the language being spoken (Weiss & Lillywhite, 1981). Articulation involves the movement of the anatomical structures as well as the production of speech sounds by such movements. Articulation results from the integrated and coordinated movements of the lips, tongue, and jaws to shape the flow of air into sounds. All of these movements must occur in coordination with the respiratory and phonatory systems. The sounds that the act of articulation produce are called **phonemes.** There are approximately 45 phonemes in the English language.

The phonetic sounds can be further classified as vowels, diphthongs, and consonants. The production of **vowels** and **diphthongs** (a combination of two vowel sounds) requires an unrestricted flow of air in the vocal tract. Vowels and diphthongs are always voiced (sounded). On the other hand, **consonants** are produced with a closed or constricted air passage. Consonants are either voiced or unvoiced.

Anatomical Structures of the Speech Mechanism

The anatomical structures of articulation include those structures involved in the production of speech.

Larynx. Voice box

Pharynx (throat cavity): Based on its relationship to the remainder of the vocal cavity, it is divided into a nasopharynx, oropharynx, and laryngopharynx

Vocal folds: Ligaments of the larynx that stretch across the interior of the larynx; they abduct and adduct.

Hard palate: Roof of the mouth/anterior portion of the palate

Soft palate: Velum/posterior portion of the palate

Tongue: Forms the floor of the palate

Maxilla: Upper jaw, holds the upper teeth

Mandible: Lower jaw, houses the lower set of teeth

Alveolar ridge: Gum sockets, covering roots of teeth

Lips: Important in producing labial sounds

Nasal Cavity: Vital for the production of sounds such as /m/, /n/, /ng/; modifies the resonance of the vocal tone

Lungs: Part of the respiratory system, necessary for inhalation and exhalation

Diaphragm: Set of muscles that separate the stomach from the thorax

Teeth: While the main function is chewing, they are important in the production of some speech sounds, such as /ð/, /f/, /v/

Trachea: Windpipe

The air tube

Each adult dental arch has sixteen teeth for a total of thirty-two teeth. The teeth are the central incisors, the lateral incisors, the canines, first and second premolars, and first, second, and third molars. The speech mechanism is shown in Figure 2.2.

Activities

- **Review some journal articles pertaining to articulation disorders and the current strategies speech-language pathologists are using to correct them.**
- **Arrange to observe a speech-language pathologist at a local school. Take note of the techniques he or she uses with students with articulation disorders.**

Summary

The speech process is a complex process, interdependent on multiple systems of the body. Each system must work in synch with the other. The central nervous, respiratory, phonatory, resonance, and articulatory systems are all involved in the act of communication. Understanding the speech process will assist you in understanding many of the problems that can occur in these systems.

References and Suggested Readings

Dickson, D., & Maue-Dickson, W. (1988). *Anatomical and physiological bases of speech*. Austin, TX: PRO-ED.

Dox, I., Melloni, B., & Eisner, G. (1989). *Melloni's illustrated medical dictionary* (2nd ed.). Baltimore, MD: Williams & Wilkins.

Geschwind, N. (1979). Specialization of the human brain. *Scientific American*. San Francisco: W. H. Freeman.

Gleason, J. B. (1989). *The development of language* (2nd ed.). Columbus, OH: Merrill.

Hedge, M. N. (1995). *Introduction to communicative disorders* (2nd ed.). Austin, TX: PRO-ED.

Hulit, L. M., & Howard, M. R. (1993). *Born to talk: An introduction to speech and language development*. New York: Macmillan.

Kahane, J. C. (1986). *Anatomy and physiology of the speech mechanism*. Austin, TX: PRO-ED.

Kurtweil, R. (1989). Beyond pattern recognition. *BYTE*, 277–288.

Munsell, P. E., Rauen, M., & Kinjo, M. (1988). Language learning and the brain: A comprehensive survey of recent conclusions. *Language Learning, 38*, 261–274.

Nicolosi, H., Harryman, E., & Krescheck, J. (1978). *Terminology of communication disorders— Speech, language, hearing*. Baltimore: Williams & Wilkins.

Sataloff, R. T. (1992, December). The human voice. *Scientific American*, 108–115.

Schneiderman, C. R. (1984). *Basic anatomy and physiology in speech and hearing*. Boston: Little, Brown.

Seikel, J. A., King, D., & Drumright, D. (1997). *Anatomy and physiology for speech and language*. San Diego: Singular Publishing Group.

Shearer, W. (1979). *Illustrated speech anatomy*. Springfield, IL: Charles C. Thomas.

Stevens, K. (1992). Theoretical aspects of speech production. *The Volta Review, 94*, 5–32.

Van Riper, C., & Erickson, R. (1996). *Speech correction: An introduction to speech pathology and audiology* (9th ed.). Boston: Allyn & Bacon.

Weiss, C., & Lillywhite, H. (1981). *Communicative disorders: Prevention and early intervention* (2nd ed.). St. Louis, MO: C. V. Mosby.

Zemlin, W. (1994). Anatomy and physiology of speech. In G. Shames, E. Wiig, & W. Secord (Eds.), *Human communication disorders* (4th ed., pp. 82–134). New York: Merrill/Macmillan.

3

Early Communication Development

Lee Cross

Chapter Objectives

After completing this chapter, the reader will be able to describe:

- Factors that influence the development of communication in young children;
- Strategies for enhancing communication development in young children;
- The normal development of communication skills for children birth through five; and
- The significance of emergent literacy in children.

- Billy is three years old, severely mentally disabled, with cerebral palsy. His skills are not far beyond those of a newborn. Cora was holding Billy in her arms talking to him, bringing her face close to his. In a soothing, adult fashion Cora told Billy about what they were going to do later that day. Cora stopped talking and stared at Billy for a long time. Pretty soon Billy started to coo while still looking at Cora. Cora didn't say a word, but continued to look into Billy's eyes. Billy stopped cooing and pretty soon Cora began to talk to him again. One more time Cora stopped talking and stared at Billy. Billy again responded by cooing.

The vignette about Cora and Billy shows the importance of the mother–child relationship in the development of communication skills. Billy's language is that of a typical young infant even though he is almost three. Cora is providing excellent intervention strategies for Billy, who is extremely delayed in all developmental areas. The cooing and turn-taking observed is a critical prelinguistic milestone in the development of communication skills.

In this chapter early communication skills and strategies to enhance their development will be discussed. It will also address:

- The normal development of communication skills for children from birth to five years;
- Factors that influence the development of speech and language in young children; and
- Strategies for enhancing language and communication for young children, particularly young children with disabilities

The development of young children between birth and the age of five is not only a critical period in the development of language but in other areas of development as well. Communicative development is related to other areas of development. The use of linguistic processes depends on attaining certain cognitive, social, and motor skills. For example, speech requires the physical growth of certain neuromuscular structures and the motor control of those structures.

It is important to know the sequence of typical early language development before problem areas are addressed that have particular implications for young children with disabilities. During the early childhood period, children master both the structure and content of language, having acquired about 2500 words in their understanding of spoken words (Bowe, 1995). The early childhood years provide the foundation for later development in all areas and are crucial in the complete development of communication skills.

> ### Reflection
> **Jimmy is standing by the swing. He runs and pulls you over to the swing and gets on the swing and sits there and looks at you. How will you respond?**

Theories of Language Development

In a discussion of theories of language development, there appears to be no coherent explanation that accounts for all the aspects of a child's development of communication competence. In fact, there is little agreement among the experts in language and communication about what theories and models hold the most promise for providing a clear picture of the communication process. Many of the models lack technical adequacy and all have their limitations in terms of providing a complete explanation for the entire process of language development in children.

However, it is useful to have an understanding of the models of language development in order to bring some order and understanding to the process. In addition, these models help educators select appropriate strategies to develop interventions and promote effective learning.

Behavioral Theory

Behaviorists focus on the observable and measurable aspects of language behavior. The meaning of the utterance is the response it produces in the listener. Behaviorists focus on the function of language, the stimuli that evoke a verbal response, and the consequence of the performance. Thus, language is a set of associations between meaning and word, word and phoneme, statement and response.

According to behavioral theory, speaking (and understanding speech) is brought under control of stimuli in the environment by reinforcement, imitation, and successive approximations to mature performance. For example, children learn that if they say, "I want a cookie," they will probably be reinforced by receiving a cookie. From a behaviorist perspective, the sequence of language acquisition proceeds through a series of environmental stimuli that are most salient at any point in time, and by the child's past experience with those stimuli (Bohannon, 1993).

Many developmental psychologists and psycholinguists criticize the behavioral theory due to the fact that it fails to explain the creative and novel use of language. However, this theory serves as the foundation of many of the language intervention techniques used today (Owens, 1988).

Psycholinguistic Theory

Linguistic approaches to language acquisition assume that the human brain contains a mental plan or structure to understand and generate language and that the plan is guided by an independent rule system. This independent rule system consists of a finite set of rules, shared by all users of the language, that produces an infinite number of comprehensible sentences. The grammatical rules are descriptions of the regularities in the language. All native speakers of a language are assumed to know the rules without being explicitly taught, although they may not be aware of the rules. Language acquisition is largely a process of children discovering the regularities in their native language. Chomsky (1957) argued that an adequate grammar must be generative or creative in order to account for the infinite sentences that speakers produce and understand.

According to Bohannon (1993) advocates of the linguistic approach believe that language is innately human, and genetic patterns of language development will be similar across different languages and cultures. The environment should play a minor role in language maturation.

The innate language component is defined as a **language acquisition device (LAD)** (Chomsky, 1965; Lenneberg, 1967). The LAD is assumed to be a specialized language processor in the brain that is activated by specific linguistic input. The exact structure of the LAD and its supporting mechanisms is a matter of great debate (Bohannon, 1993). Supposedly the LAD operates on raw linguistic data to produce the particular abstract grammar in the child's native tongue. It contains two parts: a set of rules or general principles for forming sentences and procedures for discovering how these principles are to be applied to the child's particular language.

The psycholinguistic theory is currently viewed as inadequate (Bernstein, 1993) to explain the development of the language process. The theory has contributed to the view that the child is an active and creative agent in the language development process and that there are developmental patterns that cross cultural boundaries.

Cognitive/Interactionist Theory

Interactionists: The name implies that there are many factors that affect the development of language. It is useful to explore the cognitive theory of Piaget in order to ascertain the reciprocal relationship of cognition and language. Miller (1989) points out that Piaget did not hold the common view that the source of representational thought is the ability to use words. According to Miller, Piaget thought the opposite was true, that thought is prior to language and language is the primary mode for expressing thought. Piaget did not feel that thinking is dependent on language, although language can aid cognitive development. Language is one of the tools available to enhance the cognitive system (Miller). Complex language structures are a result of the interaction between the child's current level of cognitive functioning and the immediate linguistic or nonlinguistic environment. This interactive approach is known as *constructivism* (Bohannon, 1993).

The important contributions of the cognitive interactionists to language development are pointing out the relationship between cognition and language, emphasizing the role of experience and the environment in the development of language, and focusing on a developmental perspective as a child matures and moves through stages.

Social Interactionists

The social interactionists or sociolinguists view language within its social context. Social interaction and relationships are deemed crucial because they present the child with the framework for understanding and formulating linguistic content and form (Bernstein, 1993).

This approach combines many aspects of the behavioral and linguistic positions (Bohannon, 1993). Social interactionists contend that language has a structure and follows certain rules. However, the social environment is the stimulus for communication. Language is acquired if and only if the child has reason to talk (McLean & Snyder-McLean, 1978). This theory's important contribution is in the emphasis of the social nature of language and pragmatic skills.

Each approach discussed previously describes one or more aspects of language development. As can be seen, no one theory provides a complete explanation. However, it is important to keep in mind that there are no simple explanations for a process as complex as the development of language.

> ### Reflection
>
> **You're in a circle and hold up an apple. You say to Manuel, "What color is the apple?" Manuel says, "red." What might you say to expand his verbalization? What might you say to prompt for a longer sentence?**

Prelinguistic (Preverbal) Development

The groundwork for communication development begins in the first year of life. In fact, the first few weeks of an infant's life are critical to the development of later communication skills. It is difficult to separate the development of language and communication skills from the areas of cognitive and social development. For example, when a young infant smiles on the sight of its mother, the infant is showing *recognition* (cognitive), *communicating* (language), and displaying an interest in *interacting* (social). In the early stages of development, there is an interaction between all areas of development.

Communication of Newborns

Frequently we view a newborn as the little human who lies in the crib, cries when wet, eats when hungry, and sleeps most of the time. Sometimes adults say, "After all he or she is not walking or talking, therefore, I do not have to talk much with my baby." However, during the first year of life, even before children begin to say their first words, the foundation is being laid for the development of language and communication skills. This period represents a critical time in the development of communication even before the first word appears. With the first cry, the infant is communicating intentions, needs, and desires. He or she is telling us something.

Prelinguistic development precedes the emergence of the first words (linguistic period). Infants perform purposive communication before they say their first words (Bruner, 1981). Bruner suggests that there are three categories of purposive communication during the prelinguistic stage: (1) obtaining others' assistance, (2) getting people's attention, and (3) sharing attention with others. He also observes that children use a wide variety of gestures and vocalizations to accomplish these purposes.

Prelinguistic development begins at birth with the nonverbal interchanges between the child and the parent or caregiver. Newborns have the auditory and visual skills to prepare them for early communication interactions. For example, they have the visual skills to differentiate their mothers from other women. They also begin to recognize the sound of their mother's voice and they begin to associate food and, perhaps, holding with that sound and visual image. Newborns will gaze at their mother while feeding, an early form of communication, or newborns stop crying when they hear their mother's voice. Newborns tend to track the voices and appear to distinguish them from those of other women. This is the foundation of communication development.

The cries of newborns, their facial expression, body posture, vocalizations, and even skin color communicate a great deal of information about their comfort, discomfort, interest, or readiness to engage in an interaction. Infants are communicating when their behavior gets a response from a parent or caregiver. While the intent of the behavior is not always clear in the beginning, parents quickly begin to be able to read the cues and respond in a behavioral pattern, which reinforces the infant's early communication attempts. Parents interpret the infant behavior and respond in terms of how they read the familiar infant cues. For example, when infants become fussy and start to cry around the time when they should be given their next bottle, parents know it is time to feed them.

During the second six months of life, infants begin to assert more control. They learn to communicate their intentions more clearly. The crucial factor may be the parent's responsivity and the predictability of that response (Owens, 1988). Yoder and Warren (1999) posit that intentional prelinguistic communication may be related to later language level, in part, because intentional communication elicits responsiveness, which, in turn, facilitates later language development.

Likewise, mothers quickly begin to differentiate among their infants' cries. They can tell the difference between "I'm hungry," "I'm wet," and "I want to be held" cries. During the first few months of life, babies' communication attempts are not intentional. Nevertheless, they are understood by those caring for them. This period forms the basis for conversational turn-taking and language knowledge.

Critical in the development of prelinguistic competence is parent–infant attachment. The development of communication skills is a social phenomenon as well as a linguistic set of skills, so it is critical to realize how important the bonding between an infant and its primary caregiver is to language development.

Mother–Infant Attachment.   Attachment is the strong affectional relationship between a mother and her infant. This relationship serves as the cornerstone for the social and emotional development of young children, but has a strong relationship with early communication development as well. Through the attachment between the primary caregiver and the infant, trust develops. Connor, Williamson, and Siepp (1978) offer a glimpse of the importance of the reciprocal relationship between the young child and the primary caregiver:

> The baby signals his need for some kind of caretaking by crying or fussing; the mother [caregiver] responds by picking up the child; the child responds in turn with some kind of body reaction such as cuddling. The baby's bodily adjustments signal to the mother that he is ready for the next step, be it diapering, feeding, bathing, or just cuddling and stroking. The baby responds to caregiving by quieting, which reinforces the caregiving. (p. 253)

The communication process between primary caregivers and infants continues to develop through the establishment of this trust relationship, which is based on a chain of cues and responses. The speech and language to infants is systematically modified from that used in normal conversation. The adapted speech is referred to as *motherese* or *baby talk*. *Motherese* is characterized by short utterance length and simple syntax (Owens, 1988). Mothers use facial expressions and context to communicate and convey meaning when communicating with their young children.

Blacher and Meyers (1983), in their review of attachment of families with a child with a disability, stressed that the decreased responsiveness of many infants with developmental disabilities may adversely affect attachment. Such decreased responsiveness may be characterized by delays in vocalizations, infrequent smiling and crying, and lack of eye contact (Fallen & Umansky, 1985). The infant with a disability does not give off cues that induce parental contact, so parents may avoid interacting with the infant because it is fussy, cries frequently, or is physically frail. If the parents do not receive a pleasurable response from the infant, they may reduce their interaction, which might lead to a disturbance in the attachment relationship.

Infant attachment is based on a reciprocal relationship between a parent and infant. This reciprocal relationship is based on the premise that the behavior of the infant influences the parent and vice versa (Bell, 1979). Thus, the social communication system is often negatively affected by the parent–infant relationship.

Infant Communication. Most infants begin to coo in the second month of life. Cooing involves making vowel sounds and then vowel/consonant sounds, often in response to a human face, contact, or voice (Anselmo, 1987). Smiling runs parallel to cooing and seems part of the communication process. Owens (1988) determined that infants were more likely to repeat the cooing if the adult responded verbally rather than nonverbally.

Around four months of age infants initiate communication with adults by smiling, cooing, or gurgling to attract attention. These strings of sounds are called **babbling.** Most of the vocalizations are single-syllable units of consonant–vowel or vowel–consonant. They participate in rituals and game-playing, all the while learning to take turns, to share attention, and communicate their intentions through the initiation of babbling and crying for attention (Anselmo, 1987; Rossetti, 1991). At five months, the infant is able to imitate a few general sounds, usually vowels following a vocal model (Owens, 1988).

Gestures are a form of prelinguistic behavior and precede verbal communication (Rossetti, 1991). Examples of gestures, which communicate an intent, are reaching up to indicate a request to be picked up, waving bye-bye, and nodding the head to indicate yes or no. The absence of gestural behaviors may be indicative of an impending language deficit (Rossetti, 1991).

By the sixth month, infants have the ability to reflect a full repertoire of emotions in their vocalizations such as anger, pleasure, and surprise (Owens, 1988). Infants at this stage can regulate the loudness of cry or vocalizations because of the physical changes taking place. By the end of the sixth month, infants begin to babble. Babbling includes both vowel and consonant sounds (/ma/, /bu/, /pa/) and is therefore more complex than the earlier cooing. Infants continue to babble until about a month before the use of their first meaningful words and then their babbling diminishes until they say their first word.

Strategies to Encourage Prelinguistic Communication

Parents and caretakers can encourage communication at this prelinguistic level by imitating children when they vocalize. Adults will find that infants will vocalize back and a series of turn-taking interactions can take place. It is important for parents and caretakers to talk to infants as much as possible and to read simple stories to them. Parents should begin to label objects in the environment ("Here's your bottle"), parts of the body ("Look at your little toes"), while touching their toes, and people who are continually around them ("Here comes daddy"). Or, they can say a little rhyme such as "Patty cake" while touching their hands.

The last three months of the first year in typically developing children brings a new dimension to communication development . . . the intentional use of communication. During the stage of the intentional use of communication, infants are signaling in order to have a specific preplanned effect on the behavior of others. Their behavior becomes goal-directed (Anselmo, 1987). For example they might reach for a favorite toy while vocalizing, thus signaling to the caregiver that they want the toy. The caregiver or parent, in turn, gives them a toy. The infant at this stage shows comprehension and understanding, and begins to comply with simple requests such as "Wave bye-bye."

Reflection

Sally, who is five, comes to you and says, "Me want color." What will you say?

Early Language Development

Development of Single Words

By twelve months infants recognize their own name and can follow simple motor instructions. They also react to "no" and begin using some words in the presence of a referent. Single words are used for more than naming. They are used for requesting, commenting, and inquiring. Generally, first words are family members, pets, toys, or foods. After a child acquires one word, he or she will usually use a few more within a short time and then reach a plateau. Between the end of the first year and eighteen months, infants begin to say single words, often, "mama." Single words usually refer to people and things in their environment that satisfy wants and needs. Words become symbolic and follow certain conventions.

When children are about two-and-a-half, they begin to combine two words and to increase their rate of vocabulary growth. During this time there is a decrease in the use of jargon and babbling.

By the end of the second year, children may be saying as many as 300–350 words and combining the words into sentences (Stoel-Gammon, 1998). When children first start combining words, they use those that have the most meaning for them. Language at this stage is telegraphic in that the child's word combinations only include the essential words, such as "More milk," meaning "I want more milk." or "Baby cookie," meaning "I want a cookie." Linguists have classified these early sentences into seven main categories (Anselmo, 1987):

- **Descriptions,** "Cookie gone."
- **Questions,** "Where Daddy?"
- **Possessions,** "Mine dolly."
- **Recurrence,** "More milk."
- **Agent Action,** "Doggie bite."
- **Negation and Wish,** "No go bed" and "Drink Coke."
- **Location,** "Baby here."

Roger Brown (1973), after completing a longitudinal study of the language development of young children, developed a system for classifying development using the value of **mean length of utterance (MLU).** Brown noted that there are certain characteristic periods of language development that correspond to increases in the child's average utterance length measured in morphemes. In order to compute a child's mean length of utterance, the total number of morphemes from a child's language sample divides the total number of words. Brown identified fourteen morphemes, which included two prepositions (*in, on*), two articles (*a, the*) noun inflections (possessives and plurals by adding *-s*), verb inflections (the progressive *-ing*, third person present tense, and the past tense of regular verbs, *-ed* and irregular verbs), and the primary use of the verb *be,* both as a contraction and when it cannot be contracted (*I am, I'm, or I was*). The process of acquiring these morphemes is a gradual one, and children's usage of them is sporadic until it becomes consistent (Tager-Flusberg, 1993). Owens (1988) provides the following summary of Brown's stages, the number of MLUs, the approximate age in months, and a brief description of the characteristics.

MLU	*Approximate Age*	*(Months)*	*Characteristics*
I	1.0–2.0	12–26	Linear semantic rules
II	2.0–2.5	27–30	Morphologic development
III	2.5–3.0	31–34	Sentence form development
IV	3.75–4.5	41–46	Joining of clauses
V	4.5+	47+	

As indicated, between the ages of two and two-and-a-half years, grammatical morphemes typically begin to be included. The child uses verb inflections such as *ing* and *ed* and plural forms of nouns. The child says, "There are two dogs." Sometimes these are used inappropriately. For example, the child will say "I have two foots" or "I sitted on the chair." While these grammatical structures may be used incorrectly, they are a more sophisticated stage than the earlier telegraphic speech.

Even the simplest two-word utterances show evidence of **syntax.** The child combines words to create sentences following certain rules rather than in a random fashion (Tager-Flusberg, 1993). Table 3.1 provides a summary of the development of language for children from fifteen to sixty months. These ages are approximate as development is individual and there is a large variation among young children.

Developing Simple Sentences

By the age of three, most children begin to use simple sentences, often with three to four words. The sentences contain a subject and predicate. The three-year-old is able to ask questions, give commands, and use simple declarative sentences. Most three-year-olds have mastered the vowel sounds and the consonants /p/, /m/, /h/, /n/, /w/, /b/, /k/, /g/, and /d/ (Owens, 1988). Between three and four years of age, vocabulary grows rapidly. As noted in Table 3.1, by the age of three the child has typically acquired between 900 and 1000 words. The child's expressive and receptive vocabulary expands, and by four a child typically has mastered the basic grammar of language and has acquired 1500–1600 words and is full of questions. Usually children can use one modifier or an article with a noun and most regular and irregular past tense verbs are used correctly.

Prerequisites to Language Acquisition for Young Children

Acquiring language for young children is a complex process in which systems function in an integrated fashion. In order for young children to acquire language in a normal sequence, all of the systems must work. If there is a deficit in one of the systems, the result will be a delay in the acquisition of language and the ability to communicate. An inefficient neurophysiological system, a damaged sensory system, and limited intellectual or cognitive abilities will result in delays in the acquisition of language. Table 3.2 illustrates some indicators of possible communication delays.

From the first day children are born, they experience the world, in part, based on what they hear. Communication between parents and children is largely based on the ability to verbalize and to hear. As they develop, they begin to notice sounds around them, such as the sound of someone's voice, a dog barking, a music box and so on. Later, children begin to comprehend and associate the word (symbol) labels of the people and things in the environment. They experience interactions based on communication with themselves, their peers, and adults in their family

TABLE 3.1 *Summary of Communication Skills*

Age (in months)	Skill	Age (in months)	Skill
15		36	Has 900–1000 word vocabulary
16	Points to toys, persons, animals, clothes named		Creates three–four word sentences
	Uses jargon and words in conversation		Uses simple sentence construction with subject and verb
	Has four- to six-word vocabulary		Plays with words and sounds
18	Begins to use two-word utterances		Follows two-step command
	Has approximately a twenty-word vocabulary		Talks about the present
	Identifies some body parts	48	Has 1,500–1,600-word vocabulary
	Refers to self by name		Asks many, many questions
	Sings spontaneously		Uses increasingly complex sentences
	Plays question and answer with adults		Retells stories and the simple past
21	Likes rhyming games		Understands most questions about the immediate environment
	Understands personal pronouns		Has some difficulty answering how and why
	Uses *I* and *mine*		Relies on word order for interpretation
	Pulls person to show something		
24	Has 200- to 300-word vocabulary	60	Has vocabulary of 2100–2200 words
	Names common everyday objects		Discusses feelings
	Uses short sentences		Understands *before* and *after*
	Uses some prepositions (*in, on*) and pronouns *I, me,* and *you* but not always correctly		Follows a three-step command
	Uses some verb endings (*-s, -ed, -ing*) and plural *s*		Has 90% grammar acquisition

Adapted from: Owens, R. E., Jr. (1988). Child development. In *Language development: An introduction* (2nd ed., pp. 63–103). Columbus, OH: Merrill.

and community. Often parents and others adapt their communication to the level of young children, simplifying their normal conversation style so that they will understand. So much occurs linguistically in the first five years of life that even a minor hearing loss can have a serious effect on the development of language (Fallen & Umansky, 1985).

TABLE 3.2 *Indicators of Possible Communication Delays in Young Children*

Neonates (Birth to 28 days)	Does not show startle response to a loud noise Does not look eye-to-eye when being held
One to Four Months	Does not babble Does not laugh Does not turn head in direction of a sound
Four to Eight Months	Does not babble Does not laugh Does not demonstrate an interest in new and different sounds Does not calm to primary caretaker's voice
Eight to Twelve Months	Does not obey "no" or other simple commands Does not play with sounds or make first word
Twelve to Eighteen months	Does not speak in a variety of one-word utterances Does not answer questions with "yes" or "no" or other appropriate responses
Eighteen to twenty-four months	Does not speak using a variety of two-word utterances in speech that is intelligible to people familiar with the toddler's speech Does not obey simple spoken commands unless the request is also made in gesture or other visual modes
Three Years	Does not speak in a variety of three- or four-word utterances Does not have speech that is at least occasionally intelligible to strangers Does not tell own name on request

Adapted from: Prizant, B., & Weatherby, A. M. (1993). Communication and language assessment for young children. *Infants and Young Children, 5*(4), 20–34.

Reflection

You are sitting in a circle, and you ask Johnny to point to his nose. Instead, he points to his eye. What will you do?

Vision.   The relationship of visual acuity to the development of reading and writing skills, a form of language and communication, is obvious. However, a visual impairment has an effect on language development in infancy. Adults are continually labeling objects in the environment, which enables children to organize and label their world as it is presented to them. Because visually impaired children cannot see well, it is difficult for them to see and recognize the things being discussed. Adults must use auditory and tactile clues to help children develop the conceptual understanding that parallels the language. As emphasized in Chapter 1, nonverbal elements—gestures and body language—are part of the communicative process.

Again, these aspects of communication are not available for children with visual impairment, making communication not only difficult but very different.

Cognition.   Many children with disabilities are cognitively delayed. Cognition or intelligence parallel language development. That is why many children with educational disabilities are delayed in language acquisition. The content of a child's language is dependent on what he or she is able to represent, organize, and understand in the environment (Armbruster & Klein, 1996).

Two subskills of cognition, memory and attention, directly affect language acquisition. Children must formulate a visual image in memory so that the auditory symbol used to represent the image will have a referent. Children rehearse the language they are learning both orally and to themselves, and memory plays an important part in their language rehearsal. They have to store the information and then be able to retrieve it when it is time to demonstrate comprehension or produce the correct word or words for the referent.

Attention is also critical to language development. Children must attend to and note critical features of an image or concept being learned. In addition, they must also attend to the word order, what is being said, and the sounds involved in making words.

Physical.   The central nervous system of children must be intact. Speech and language development depends on the ability not only to receive incoming auditory information but also to process, organize, retrieve, and store that information. Motor skills are also important in the development of communication skills. The production of speech sounds involves the careful coordination of the muscles involved in the movement of the tongue, lips, jaw, velum, larynx, and muscles of respiration. For children with motor impairments such as cerebral palsy, the production of speech is very difficult.

Structural abnormalities such as craniofacial deformities interfere with speech development. For example, if there is a deviant mouth structure that precludes placing the tongue and teeth in the correct relationship to one another, the child will have difficulty saying /th/ in the words *this* or *think.* Children with a cleft palate may speak with a nasal voice, which makes speech almost unintelligible.

Environmental.   Some children grow and develop in an environment where language and communication are not encouraged. Parents sometimes assume that it is not important to talk to a baby or young child and carry on conversation because they are too little and can't talk back. Consequently, they are left in their cribs without any interaction. Sometimes parents are stressed because of the demands of their own lives and interacting with a young child is a low priority. Many parents view their children, when they respond to an adult, as being "sassy" and encourage them to sit down and be quiet. This behavior on the part of the caregiver does not encourage the development of communication skills. Some homes lack books and play materials that can serve as vehicles for communication development. Even in homes where there are books or toys, sometimes children are sent off to play by themselves. Because communication is based on social interaction, children are not given an opportunity to interact with others using the toys and books.

Strategies to Facilitate the Development of Communication Skills

Communication skills are a critical developmental area for young children. It is important that parents and educators are aware of some strategies for facilitating communication skills in young children with and without disabilities. The following discussion will provide a sampling of strategies to enhance communication skills. These strategies may be useful for parents as well as teachers and caregivers.

Facilitation Strategies Should Occur in the Natural Environment and Be Functional

The facilitation of communication skills should be integrated into all the daily activities of children whether at home or in day-care centers, preschool programs or early intervention programs. It is not terribly effective to provide communication training in isolation. Even young children who receive individual therapy need opportunities for communication in the context of everyday activities. Children who receive communication therapy often fail to generalize the target behaviors to everyday activities, so these individual sessions fail to fully remediate the problem or deficits (Roberts, Bailey, & Nychka, 1991).

A Communication-Rich Environment Facilitates the Development of Communication Skills. In order for communication skills to develop, children need to talk and listen. Conversation needs to be encouraged. Certainly books and toys provide vehicles for communication because children enjoy talking about things that they are interested in. However, a language-rich environment also includes adults who talk with children during the routine activities such as during bath time, at meals, and while driving in the car. A communication-rich environment includes adults who encourage conversation and take time to listen to children and ask them questions rather than tell them to go away and play.

It has also been suggested that sometimes it is effective to modify the environment to encourage communication. For example, a caregiver might put a toy out of reach in order to encourage the child to request the toy. Only after the child attempts to communicate is the child given the toy to play with. If a child appears particularly thirsty and gulps down a first cup of milk and appears to want more, the caregiver might say, "Tell me you want more milk." Say, "I want more milk." This says to the child "You must use language to communicate your wants," and "There is a cause and effect relationship between what I want and my communication."

Reflection

Following are some situations that require adults to provide selected language facilitation strategies. Please write or discuss in small groups what you should say based on the previous discussion in this chapter.

- Annie is playing with blocks. She is stacking blocks on top of each other. What might you say to her to describe what she is doing? What might you ask her that will facilitate expressive language? What might you say to her to reflect her feelings?
- Tony is sitting at the table and looks at the plate of cookies. He reaches for a cookie. What might you say to prompt him to ask for a cookie?
- Danielle is painting at the easel with blue and green paints. What might you say to her to describe what she is doing? What might you say to her to encourage her to use expressive language?

Responding to Communication Attempts.   Caregivers of young children with disabilities often become discouraged due to the noninteractive nature of some children with disabilities. Responding to any communication attempt, particularly if the child initiates the attempt to communicate, even if unintelligible, is crucial to supporting the development of communicative abilities (Roberts, Bailey, & Nychka, 1991).

Prompting and Cueing.   Children who are reluctant to respond to a question or a communication attempt by another child will benefit from a prompt or cue. Prompts or cues may be verbal or physical. A prompt or cue offers the child a form of a response. A prompt may even be in the form of offering the child choices. For example, if Natasha asked Raphael what he wants to play and Raphael fails to answer, an adult might say, "Do you want to play with the blocks or with the trucks?" After Raphael responds, the adult might say, "Raphael, tell Natasha you want to play blocks." In this situation, the adult is prompting Raphael to make a communication response. The adult is not doing the talking for him, but giving Raphael the words to engage in a communication interaction.

Help Children Attend in Conversation.   To attend in conversation, children must have a number of skills, including making eye contact, listening carefully to the speaker, and moving to position themselves at a distance, which makes conversation easy. Sometimes children need to be prompted to attend. For example, an adult might say, "Johnny look at me," if the adult is going to say something, or "Listen to Susie, she just asked you a question." Sometimes prompts might be verbal or physical. Taking a child's face and gently turning him or her toward the speaker while saying "Look" is helpful in encouraging attending behavior. Positioning oneself at the child's level by stooping down or sitting on a low chair or on the floor is also helpful in encouraging attending behavior. A big person towering over them can easily overwhelm children.

Describing Events.   Caretakers should describe events occurring around the child. This builds receptive language and provides the child with good language models. A parent may comment to his child while in the kitchen by saying, "I'm going to make dinner now. I have to peel the potatoes. I'm getting the knife and peeling the potatoes." When an adult describes or comments it does not require a response from the child. The activities, which are being described, should be concrete and tied to the current environment and context of the child. The sentences should be short and simple based on the developmental level of the child.

Repeat Child's Response.   An effective facilitation strategy is to repeat what the child says directly. For example an adult asks Latesha, "What color is an apple?" Latesha responds by saying, "Red." The adult responds by saying, "Red." Then the adult might ask another question. Repeating a child's response communicates to the child the importance of communication and reinforces the response.

Expanding Children's Responses.   In expanding or elaborating on the child's response the adult takes the response of the child and adds words or phrases. Expansions provide a model for the child and at the same time confirm that the message the child gave was understood and valued (Chapman, 1988). For example, if the child says, "want cookie," the caregiver might respond by saying "Judy wants a cookie" as she gives Judy a cookie. This interaction confirms Judy's intent, yet at the same time expands the sentence and provides a model for the child. It is important when expanding responses that only one or two words are added to the child's original sentence. If the expansion is too complex, the child will ignore the adult response. Expansions appear to be most effective when the child is producing two- and three-word utterances (Fey, 1986; McDade & Varnedoe, 1987; Reike & Lewis, 1984) and are particularly important for young children with disabilities.

Prompting Communication to Replace Undesirable Behavior.   Often when preschool children don't have the language to communicate their needs and desires, they respond through inappropriate behavior such as grabbing a toy or hitting another child. It has been suggested that caregivers identify the intent of the undesirable behavior and provide the language to replace that behavior. For example, if a child grabs another child's truck, the caregiver might say, "José, ask Natasha if you can play with the truck." Reike and Lewis (1984) note that inappropriate behaviors should be replaced with appropriate communication responses rather than totally eliminating the negative behavior.

Giving the Child More Time.   Often children need time to respond. Adults frequently jump in too quickly and talk for the child. This adult behavior discourages any communication attempt on the part of the child. It says to the child, if I don't talk someone else will. Why should I bother?

Reflection

You are reading the story of the "Three Little Pigs." You say to Billy, "Tell me something about the first little pig." Billy says, "Sticks." What will you say?

Emergent Literacy

I would be remiss in not including a discussion of emergent literacy in a chapter about communication and young children. Language and literacy are simultaneously learned and interrelated (Koppenhaver, Pierce, Steelman, & Yoder, 1995).

Vygostsky (1978) defines literacy as part of a unified historical line of the development of symbolism from speech, through play and drawing to reading and writing. Learning to read requires numerous abilities, several of which are acquired before a child begins school.

Emergent literacy is a concept that has gained interest in recent years. Professionals in child development no longer believe that reading is a process that begins at five or six, but that it begins in infancy when a parent first reads to their young children and they come into contact with print. Literacy is no longer thought of as totally a cognitive skill but as a complex socio-psycholinguistic activity (Teale & Sulzby, 1989). Emergent literacy refers to the first signs of abilities and knowledge with regard to written language, the period between birth and the time when children conventionally read and write (Sulzby & Teale, 1991).

Frequent contact with written language provides young children an opportunity to develop a positive attitude toward reading and writing (Saint-Laurent, Giasson, & Couture, 1997). Through listening to stories, young children will learn to enjoy literature and be motivated to read themselves. They will also develop a concept of print, which is vital to their success in early reading (Shearer & Homan, 1994). When children understand that print carries a message, they have developed the first and most important emergent literacy concept. According to Koppenhaver, Coleman, Kalman, and Yoder (1991), the functions of literacy are as integral to literacy learning as the forms. A fundamental emergent literacy concept is that reading and writing are purposeful activities and are done for reasons (functions). Children learn from observation that reading and writing through various forms help us do important things in our lives (Wolery & Wolery, 1992).

Young children gain an understanding and an awareness of print when they are read to, when their parents point out logos and signs on television or when riding in the car, when they see their mother using a written list in the grocery store, when they view their parents writing and reading letters from relatives and friends, or as they watch their older brothers and sisters write out their homework.

Directional concepts related to reading and writing are important emergent literacy skills (Clay, 1991), for example, when we read, we read from the top to the bottom of the page and we also read a page from left to right. In addition, young children exposed to experiences with print develop a sense of word and letter boundaries (Clay, 1991) in that they begin to identify that individual letters are part of words.

Another important emergent literacy principle according to Koppenhaver and colleagues (1991) is that young children gain literacy skills through active engagement with their world. Literacy skill acquisition is not a passive process, but a process whereby young children are actively engaged through pointing to pictures when being read a story, asking or answering question about a book they are looking at, talking about pictures they are drawing, or noticing letters and words on a cereal box or soup can.

In conclusion, during the early childhood period children are developing critical preliteracy skills that will contribute to their abilities to read and write. Speaking, listening, reading, and writing are acquired and refined concurrently (Koppenhaver et al., 1991). The child's environment, both human and physical, is critical in the development of emergent literacy. The literacy-rich environment must include materials such as books, letter blocks, paper and pencils, and so forth, opportunities to explore the materials, and interaction with adults (parents or teachers).

Reflection

Jimmy has just pushed Sammy off the tricycle and takes it and starts to ride it. Sammy is on the ground crying. What will you say to Jimmy?

Summary

Clearly, the early development of communication skills is critical for young children. These skills begin with the newborn and continue during the first five years. By five the child has the basic structure of language and has acquired a vocabulary of two thousand or more words.

Adults and primary caregivers can use many different strategies to facilitate early communication development. These strategies include focusing on functional skills within the natural environment, encouraging communication, responding to communication attempts, prompting and cueing, helping children attend, describing events, expanding a child's responses, and giving children time and opportunity to communicate.

References and Suggested Readings

Anselmo, S. (1987). *Early childhood development: Prenatal through age eight.* New York: Macmillan.

Armbruster, V. B., and Klein, M. D. (1996). Nurturing communication skills. In R. Cook, A. Tessier, & M. D. Klein (Eds.), *Adapting early childhood* curricula for children in inclusive settings (4th ed., pp. 312–36). Columbus, OH: Merrill.

Bell, R. J. (1979). Parent, child, and reciprocal influences. *American Psychologist, 34,* 821–826.

Bernstein, D. K. (1993). The nature of language and its disorders. In D. K. Bernstein & E. Tiegerman (Eds.), *Language and communication disorders in children* (3rd ed., pp. 2–22). New York: Macmillan.

Blacher, J., & Meyers, C. E. (1983). A review of attachment formation and disorders of handicapped children. *American Journal of Mental Deficiency, 87,* 359–371.

Bohannon, J. N., III. (1993). Theoretical approaches to language acquisition. In J. B. Gleason (Ed.), *The development of language* (3rd ed., pp. 239–297). New York: Macmillan.

Bowe, F. G. (1995). *Birth to five: Early childhood special education.* New York: Delmar.

Brown, R. (1973). *The first language: The early stages.* Cambridge, MA: Harvard University Press.

Bruner, J. (1981). The social context of language acquisition. *Language and Communication, 1,* 155–178.

Chapman, R. S. (1988). Language acquisition in the child. In N. J. Lass, L. V. McReynolds, J. L. Northern, & D. E. Yoder (Eds.), *Handbook of speech, language, pathology and audiology* (pp. 219–233). Hillsdale, NJ: Lawrence Erlbaum.

Chomsky, N. (1957). *Syntactic structures.* The Hague: Mouton.

Chomsky, N. (1965). *Aspects of the theory of syntax.* Cambridge: MA: MIT Press.

Clay, M. M. (1991). *Reading: Becoming literate* (3rd ed.). Auckland, New Zealand: Heinemann.

Connor, F. P., Williamson, G. G., and Siepp, J. M. (1978). *Program guide for infants and toddlers with neuromotor and other developmental disabilities.* New York: Teachers College Press.

Fallen, N. H., & Umansky, W. (1985). *Young children with special needs.* Columbus, OH:Merrill.

Fey, M. (1986). *Language intervention with young children.* San Diego: College-Hill Press.

Koppenhaver, D. A., Coleman, P. P., Kalman, S. L., & Yoder, D. E. (1991). The implications of emergent literacy research for children with developmental disabilities. *American Journal of Speech-Language Pathology, 1*(1), 38–44.

Koppenhaver, D. A., Pierce, P. L., Steelman, J. D., & Yoder, D. E. (1995). Contexts of early literacy intervention for children with developmental disabilities. In M. E. Fey, J. Windsor, & S. F. Warren (Vol. Eds.), *Language intervention:* Preschool through the elementary years, Vol. 5 (pp. 241–274). Baltimore. Paul H. Brooks.

Kuhl, P. K. (1985). Categorization of speech by infants. In J. Mehler & R. Fox (Eds.), *Neonate cognition: Beyond the blooming buzzing confusion* (pp. 231–262). Hillsdale, NJ: Lawrence Earlbaum.

Lenneberg, E. (1967). *Biological foundations of language.* New York: Wiley.

McDade, H. L., & Varnedoe, D. R. (1987). Training parents to be language facilitators. *Topics in Language Disorders, 7,* 19–30.

McLean, J., & Snyder-McLean, L. (1978). *A transactional approach to early language training.* Columbus, OH: Merrill.

Miller, P. H. (1989). *Theories of developmental psychology* (2nd ed.). New York: W. H. Freeman.

Owens, R. E., Jr. (1988). *Language development. An introduction* (2nd ed.). Columbus, OH:Merrill.

Prizant, B., & Bailey, D. (1992). Facilitating the acquisition and use of communication skills. In D. Bailey and M. Worley (Eds.), *Teaching infants and preschoolers with disabilities* (2nd ed., pp. 291–361). Columbus, OH: Merrill.

Prizant, B., & Weatherby, A. M. (1993). Communication and language assessment for young children. *Infants and Young Children, 5*(4), 20–34.

Reike, J., & Lewis, J. (1984). Preschool intervention strategies: The communication base. *Topics in Language Disorders, 5,* 41–57.

Roberts, J. E., Bailey, D. B., & Nychka, H. B. (1991). Teachers' use of strategies to facilitate the communication of preschool children with disabilities. *Journal of Early Intervention, 15,* 358–376.

Rosetti, L. (1991). Social and communication development in infancy. In S. Raver (Ed.), *Strategies for teaching at-risk and handicapped infants and toddlers: A transdisciplinary approach* (pp. 105–136). New York: Macmillan.

Saint-Laurent, L., Giasson, J., Couture, C. (1997). Parents + children + reading activities = emergent literacy. *TEACHING Exceptional Children, 30*(2), 52–56.

Shearer, A. P., & Homan, S. P. (1994). *Linking reading assessment to instruction: An application worktext for elementary classroom teachers.* New York: St. Martin's Press.

Stoel-Gammon, C. (1998). Role of babbling and phonology in prelinguistic development. In A. M. Wetherby, S. F. Warren, & J. Reichle (Eds.), *Transitions in prelinguistic communication* (pp. 87–110). Baltimore, MD: Paul H. Brookes.

Sulzby, E., & Teale, W. (1991). Emergent literacy. In R. Barr, M. L. Kamil, P. Mosenthal, & D. Pearson (Eds.), *Handbook of reading research* (Vol. 2, pp. 727–757). New York: Longman.

Tager-Flusberg, H. (1993). Putting words together: Morphology and syntax in the preschool years. In J. Berko Gleason (Ed.), *The development of language* (3rd ed., pp. 151–194). New York: Macmillan.

Teale, W. H., & Sulzby, E. (1989). Emergent literacy: New perspectives. In D. S. Strickland & L. M. Morrow (Eds.), *Emerging literacy: Young children learn to read and write.* Newark, DE: International Reading Association.

Vygostky, L. S. (1978). *Mind in society: The development of higher psychological processes.* Cambridge, MA: Harvard University Press.

Wolery, M., & Wolery, R. A. (1992). Promoting functional cognitive skills. In D. B. Bailey & M. Wolery (Eds.), *Teaching infants and preschoolers with disabilities* (2nd ed., pp. 521–572). New York: Merrill.

Yoder, P. J., & Warren, S. F. (1999). Maternal responsivity mediates the relationship between prelinguistic intentional communication and later language. *Journal of Early Intervention, 22,* 126–136.

The Development of Language Skills in School-Age Children

Lee Cross

Chapter Objectives _____

On completion of this chapter, the reader will be able to:

- Discuss the development of oral language, both receptive and expressive, through the school years;
- Use the three components of language: form (phonology, morphology, and syntax), content (semantics), and use (pragmatics) as the conceptual framework.

Components of Language

- Marilyn Nippold (1992) tells an incident about Kenny, a seven-year-old, who was discussing the story of "The Three Little Pigs" with his speech and language clinician, using the picture book. The dialogue between the two was as follows:

   Clinician: Tell me about this little pig, Kenny. (Clinician points to picture of pig, including a brick house.)

   Kenny: um . . . um . . . something . . . uh . . . um . . . um . . . something . . . made of . . . um . . . um . . . and somebody bricked (built) that house . . . brick house . . . /
   I'm saying . . . something and somebody brick (built) this house/
   It's . . . uh . . . it's the . . . uh . . . let see the second pig . . . bricked (built) the house . . . /

I think it's the second house . . . /
I gotta find the second pig . . . (p. 1).

The vignette illustrates a child with a word-finding disorder. **Word finding** is the ability to store and retrieve words and messages. This is a language skill that school-age students can usually do with little effort, particularly with the aid of pictures. Typically, students can retrieve the words they need to retell a story they have heard over and over again.

As we are well aware, the development of language is a complex process. The early childhood period is a time of rapid skill development. While the preschool period is critical in language development, the school years are equally important. Throughout the school-age years, there is an increase in the size and complexity of the child's linguistic repertoire as well as in the use of language (Owens, 1988). The school-age period increases with importance as we realize the language requirements for a student to be successful in school. Not only do students have to become competent in the abstract uses of language through reading and writing, but they have to become good listeners and oral communicators. Children acquire not only more complex forms of language but more complex uses. Table 4.1 presents an overview of some of the important milestones of the language development of school-age children.

Language is a complex combination of three major components: form, content, and use (Bloom & Lahey, 1975). As previously mentioned, *language* refers to "a code whereby ideas about the world are expressed through a conventional system of arbitrary signals for communication." (Lahey, 1988, p. 2). Oral language involves both speaking and listening, whereas written language involves reading and writing at both the expressive and receptive level. A person's ability to understand information is referred to as comprehension or **receptive language** (listening and reading). The ability to produce information is **expressive language** (oral expression and writing). In oral language, both speaking and listening are important for the communication process. A listener must use receptive language and comprehension to understand a message. A speaker must use the symbols of language (words and sounds) to communicate ideas and message. This chapter will discuss the oral language, both receptive and expressive, using the three components of language: form (phonology, morphology, and syntax), content (semantics), and content (pragmatics) as the framework. Table 4.2 (p. 59) summarizes the components of language and the levels.

Form

Form refers to the structure and sound of language. Form is further divided into phonology, morphology, and syntax.

TABLE 4.1   *Summary of School-Age Students' Language Development*

Age	Form	Content	Use
5	Syntax/Morphology: Produces short passives		Uses mostly direct requests; repeats for repair; begins to use gender topics
6	Phonology: Identifies syllables; Morphology: Acquires rule for plural; comprehends imperative commands, and the suffix *-er* Syntax: Uses *many* with plural nouns		Responds to indirect hints; repeats with elaboration with repair; uses adverbs such as *now, then, so, though*
7	Phonology: Is able to manipulate sound units to rhyme or produce stems; recognizes unacceptable sound sequence Syntax: Comprehends *because*; follows adult ordering of adjectives	Uses left/right and front/back	Uses and understands most terms that indicate the process of using the speaker's perspective as a reference (examples include *this, that, me,* and *you*)
8	Phonology: Is able to produce all English sounds Syntax: Uses full passives (80% of the children)		Sustains concrete topics; begins considering others' intentions
9		Can shift word association from a syntactic to semantic basis	Sustains topics through several turns Addresses perceived source of breakdown in repair
10	Syntax: Comprehends and uses *ask*		
11	Syntax: Comprehends *if* and *though* Uses *much* with mass nouns	Creates abstract definitions; uses conventional form definitions; understands psychological states described with physical terms	Sustains abstract topic

(continued)

TABLE 4.1   *Continued*

Age	Form	Content	Use
12	Phonology: Uses stress contrasts		Uses adverbial conjuncts—*otherwise, anyway, therefore,* and *however* Disjoins *really* and *probably*
13–15	Syntax: Comprehends embedding of all types	Comprehends proverbs Comprehends *unless* Comprehends *at* used for temporal relations	
16–18	Phonology: Uses vowel-shifting rules (divine/divinity)		Uses sarcasm and double meanings Makes deliberate use of metaphors Knows partner's perspective and knowledge differ from own

Adapted from Owens, R. E. (1988). *Language development: An introduction* (2nd ed., pp. 324–325). Columbus, OH: Merrill.

Phonology.   By age eight, according to Owens (1988), a child can produce all of the sounds in English, although sounds in longer words and blends may still be difficult. Owens also notes that vowels are acquired by age three, whereas consonant clusters and blends are not acquired until seven or eight.

There is an increasing body of research documenting the relationship between delays in reading and spelling and weaknesses in phonemic awareness (MacDonald & Cornwall, 1995; Torgesen, Wagner, & Rashotte, 1994). Phonological awareness is the process of breaking down words presented auditorily into their individual sounds. Five-year-olds are typically proficient at rhyming, segmenting words into individual sounds, identifying sounds at the beginning and ending of words, and sound blending (Smith, 1998). According to Smith, by the end of first grade children should be able to separate words into their individual sounds, split syllables, delete sounds from words, substitute sounds, and reverse sounds.

Morphology.   Morphology focuses on the rule system that governs the structure of words and word forms. Elementary students learn the various inflectional endings, suffixes, and prefixes. Developmentally, inflectional endings are the easiest to learn, followed by suffixes, and then prefixes (Owens, 1995). Inflectional endings can be taught through conversation and modeling; prefixes and suffixes are usually taught through more formal instruction in both oral and written form (Bos & Vaughn, 1998).

Syntax.   Syntax refers to the order of words in a sentence and the rules for determining the order. An important aspect of language for school-age children is

TABLE 4.2   *Components and Levels of Language*

Component	Definition	Receptive Level	Expressive Level
Form	*Phonology*: The sound system of the language and the rules that govern the sound combinations.	Discrimination of the speech sounds	Articulation of speech sounds
	Morphology: The rule system that governs the construction of word forms from the basic elements of meaning.	Understanding the grammatical structure of words	Use of grammar in words
	Syntax: The rule system governing the order of words to form sentences and the relationships among the elements in a sentence.	Understanding the phrases and sentences	Use of grammar in phrases and sentences
Content	*Semantics*: The psycholinguistic system that patterns the content and meanings of words in sentences.	Understanding of word meanings and word relationships	Use of word meanings and relationships
Use	*Pragmatics*: The sociolinguistic system that patterns the use of language in communication that may be expressed motorically or verbally.	Understanding the context of language and the cues	Use of language in context

Source: From *Students with Learning Disabilities* (5th ed., p. 422), by C. D. Mercer, 1997, Upper Saddle River, NJ: Merrill/Prentice-Hall.

syntactic development (Scott & Stokes, 1995). Syntax is a focus in elementary classrooms in both writing and speaking. One of the primary foci is an awareness of the sentence as a primary linguistic unit. However, there are problems with isolating syntax from discourse and semantics (Scott, 1995). As student's get older they develop more complex sentence structures. By age six, children understand the imperative. After age seven, they have mastered comprehension of irregular noun and verb agreement, conjunctions, passive sentences, and several verb tenses such as past and perfect participles (Wood, 1976; Owens, 1988). Average sentence length matches chronological age in oral discourse until around nine, when the growth ceases (Bos & Vaughn, 1998). By adolescence, students' conversational utterances average ten to twelve words (Scott & Stokes).

Content

Content, also referred to as semantics, refers to the ideas or concepts one is communicating. The content of language refers to the meaning, both what is expressed and what is received. Much of what we teach in school focuses on content. The content may be shapes for younger children or the causes of the Civil War for older children. The focus is ideas, the relationship between and among ideas and the vocabulary that labels the ideas (Bos & Vaughn, 1998).

School-age students increase the size of their vocabularies and their abilities to understand and talk about abstract concepts and ideas. Vocabulary development involves the acquisition of new words and new meanings and the establishment of links between them (Pease, Gleason, & Pan, 1993). By six years, children are able to comprehend between 20,000 and 24,000 words and, by twelve, their vocabulary has doubled to about 50,000 or more words (Owens, 1988). The size of a child's vocabulary depends, in part, on the experiences and words to which the child is exposed. School provides students an opportunity to listen, learn, and read about ideas and concepts in science, social studies, literature, and math, thus providing the context for expanding their vocabularies. New words are continually added to their lexicons. To learn a new word meaning, a child must learn how her or his language community has grouped and labeled the various aspects of an experience. In the beginning, children develop their vocabulary based on their experience and the context in which the words are encountered. For example, a preschool child may have the concept of "plant" as something green that grows in the dirt. However, a student in an upper elementary grade would define *plant* as not only something green that grows, but something that needs soil, oxygen, and sun in order to grow. In addition, the older student would differentiate between the types of things that grow such as vegetables, flowers, trees, and so on. An older student might expand the definition to include activities that require verbs such as sowing seeds or depositing the living thing in the soil. The older student might also define *plant* with its slang meaning, "to hoax or trick or frame." Thus, older students have developed multiple meanings of words and concepts and expanded their vocabulary based on not only their own experiences but new information they have acquired through their peers, home and family, and community and school. In addition, students increase their vocabulary through mediums such as reading and television.

Activities

Ask two children of different ages to define the terms in *italic* in the following sentences. Compare the children's responses.

- Mr. Jones was a painter. He got a *blup* and opened the paint and began to stir it before he dipped his brush in to begin painting the house. What do you think a *blup* is and what does it look like?
- The boys sat on the steps, opened the bag, got out a *grom,* and took a big bite and wiped the crumbs off their face as they took a drink of their

water. One of the boys said, "Boy this was good. I think I will have my mother make some more." What do you think a *grom* is?
- The *costis* were red and yellow. Butterflies were hovering around the *costi* and you could smell their fragrance a block away. What are *costis*?

Fast Mapping.   One way that children appear to learn new words is through a process known as fast mapping or quick incidental learning (Dollaghan, 1985, 1987; Heibeck & Markman, 1987). Children develop a meaning of a word that they don't know, based on a single exposure to the word used in a specific context. This first meaning may or may not be completely accurate. It does, however, create a basis for further refinement as additional experiences with the word in context occur.

Vocabulary development is based on the addition of new elements of meaning and reorganization of known elements (Pease et al., 1993). Growth in word knowledge results in a larger storage capacity and improves throughout childhood (Nippold, 1992). This growth occurs not only by adding new words but also by expanding the meanings of existing words and forming associations between them (Nippold, 1988).

Figurative Language.   The school-age child, as shown in Table 4.1, begins to develop the ability to understand and use figurative language. Figurative language uses words creatively, rather than literally, to create an imaginative or emotional impression, and includes the use of metaphors (*The man had fire in his eyes*) and similes (*She was mad as a hornet*). Figurative language also includes the use of idioms such as *strike a bargain*. Children in the early elementary grades tend to interpret figures of speech quite literally as they are still in the concrete operational stage (Owens, 1988). It is not until the later elementary grades that children are able to understand and use figurative language in clarifying meaning and problem-solving (Owens, 1988; Pease et. al., 1993).

Activities

Have students of different ages, (six, nine, and twelve preferably) explain the following figures of speech. Read the figure of speech and ask each child what it means. Write down each child's response and then compare the responses of the younger with the older students.

- a. The teacher asked the student a question and then the student answered. The teacher said, "Good John, you hit the nail on the head."
- b. The little boy stopped an old man and asked him how old he was. The man replied, "I am as old as the hills."
- c. It started raining and Ms. Jones looked out the window and said, "It's raining cats and dogs."

Word Finding.   This chapter began with a vignette about Kenny, a seven-year-old with word-finding deficits. Word finding is the ability to store and retrieve words, thoughts, and a sequence of events. Word-finding ability is directly related to normal information storage and retrieval process. Storage is the availability of information in memory, whereas retrieval is accessibility of that information or, in this case, words (Kobasigawa, 1977). Every item in memory has storage strength and retrieval strength. Growth in storage and retrieval is directly related to opportunities to study an item and retrieve it from memory. The human capacity for storage is unlimited (Bjork & Bjork, 1992).

According to Nippold (1988), retrieval of words and information is dependent on four critical factors: "(1) presence of cues, (2) frequency with which an item is retrieved, (3) competition with other items in the memory, and (4) recency of learning" (p. 2). Successful word finding requires that words be adequately stored in memory and easily retrievable to the speaker (Nippold, 1992). Retrieval improves as words are used with greater accuracy and speed and as strategies to facilitate recall are used more frequently and efficiently.

Some of the educational implications for students' word finding abilities are in activities such as oral presentations, exams with time limitations, filling-in-the-blank activities, writing on a particular topic, and construction of narratives. Word-finding abilities are directly related to the development of skills in reading (McGregor & Leonard, 1995).

Use

Once children begin school, they experience a great deal of developmental growth in the area of use or pragmatics (Bos & Vaughn, 1998; Nippold, 1993; Owens, 1995). Communication serves a variety of functions. A basic assumption for the communication process to be effective is that both the speaker and listener use the same code and know the same rules of language. Listening and oral expression during the school years have a variety of functions. Table 4.3 lists some of the functions. As can be seen, oral expression and listening serve a variety of functions in the classroom and are critical to learning and social interaction.

Wells (1973), as cited in Wiig & Semel (1984), categorized communication in relation to the parameters that control the intents and forms used. This categorization system has been used in the development of language assessment and intervention strategies. It provides a useful framework for understanding pragmatics. Within the system, communication acts are categorized within each of the major functions of communication, **ritualizing, informing, controlling, feeling,** and **imagining.**

The ritualizing function includes the social amenities or customs within a specific culture such as greeting, apologizing, and regulating turn-taking in games or talking on the telephone. There is a great deal of comfort in this form of communication as it is predictable and often part of the routine in a classroom or in social interactions.

TABLE 4.3   *Sampling of Communication Functions for School-Age Children*

- Listens to directions
- Gains new information, as in a lecture
- Presents new information
- Role-plays
- Expresses emotions and feelings
- Interacts with peers
- Shares information about self
- Selects different forms for oral communication based on the age, status, and reactions of the listeners
- Tells and listens to jokes and funny stories
- Listens to music
- Interviews for a part-time job
- Asks for help, assistance, or information
- Persuades others
- Requests clarification of information
- Introduces people
- Greets and says farewell to others
- Participates in classroom discussions and dialogues

The informing function of communication includes acts of sharing or exchanging information. It is frequently used in the classroom when the teacher requests the student to retell a story or answer a question during classroom discussions, the speaker must select the appropriate words to convey the ideas or content. In addition, the speaker must keep in mind the background of the listener and the contextual demands of the situation.

When speakers are trying to influence and control their listener's behavior, they are using the controlling function of language. Persuading and commanding are part of the controlling. They must be aware of not only the context, but the age and status of the listener. Controlling speech acts can be direct or indirect. It is important that the speaker is able to take the perspective of the listener in determining the directness of the communication. The ability to determine the appropriate directness increases with age.

The feeling function of communication is the expression or response to feelings and or attitudes. This function is related to the sharing of feelings and emotions or asking speakers about their feelings and attitudes. The expression of feelings and emotions can be very direct and nonintentional or intentional and indirect. A speaker's emotional state, personality, and the relationship with the listener influence the intensity conveyed in the communication act.

The imagining function places the speaker–listener in a creative or imaginary situation. This function is realized every time we role-play, tell a story, tell a lie, or speculate.

Social Function.   The ability to communicate for social purposes is critical for school-age children. Social interaction is essential for the development of friendships, relationships with adults such as teachers, parents, and other adults in the child's community, and later for older students the relationship with employers and clients or customers. Language skills are an integral part of interpersonal interactions. As Windsor (1995) attests, language acts as a major medium of social interactions and the appropriate use of it is a social skill. Language development is integral to the development of social skills, not a completely independent process (Gallagher, 1991). Cognition, as well as language, is also involved in the development of social relationships.

Some of the important language skills involved in social relationships for school-age children include asking peers to join a group, giving and receiving compliments, responding to social pleasantries (i.e., How are you?), pretending and role-playing, interacting with parents and siblings, dealing with conflicts with peers, and asking for help or assistance. For older students, certainly, the same skills are important when interviewing for a job, asking for a date, telling jokes or funny stories, gossiping with friends, negotiating issues with peers, conveying and repairing misunderstandings, interacting with teachers, carrying on conversations with friends as well as strangers, and making an apology.

Between the ages of four and eight, children make extensive gains in strategies for gaining attention, using persuasion, and making conversational repairs (Warren & McCloskey, 1993). Even though children may detect an ambiguous or inadequate message, they often fail to inform the speaker of the communication breakdown. Children may respond to inadequate messages nonverbally, but fail to provide verbal indicators of the breakdown. As the child becomes more verbally competent, he or she may assist the speaker in providing more salient messages.

When in the role of speaker, school-age children begin acquiring the ability to adjust their message to the listener. This is a complex process that has linguistic, social, and cognitive demands. They must not only have the conceptual knowledge but must also be able to adjust the communication to match the listener characteristics. Children are often only partially aware of the listener's perspective in the communication process and may not know how to adequately repair the breakdown. These abilities gradually improve over time, possibly even into adulthood, increasing the range of register variations at the speaker's command (Warren & McCloskey, 1993).

Narratives.   The ability to narrate stories underlies both social and academic development (Trousdale, 1990). When narrating stories, the child is expected to use language for an extended period, to include introductory and closing statements, to present the events in an orderly sequence, and to maintain a monologue for a relatively passive listener (Roth & Spekman, 1986). Classroom narratives support both receptive (listening and reading) and expressive (speaking and writing) language skills (Peck, 1989; Evans & Strong, 1996). Language strategies associated with written language become evident in the emerging narrative abilities of children (Dickinson, Wolf, & Stotsky, 1993). There is also evidence that the narrative discourse skills of students is directly linked to their ability to read. Students with reading delays have difficulty with the recall and production demands of narratives (Dickinson et al., 1993).

Telling stories is a social as well as a cognitive act. The use of connectives in narrative illustrates the social and cognitive skills involved in storytelling (Dickinson et al., 1993). Connectives in the narratives of older children serve not only a content (semantic) function, but a use/social function as well. The connectives (e.g., *but, because,* and *then*) inform the listener of upcoming events and the relationship between events in the narrative.

Metalinguistic Awareness. As children grow older, they develop metalinguistic awareness. **Metalinguistic awareness** is the ability to reflect on language as a decontextualized object (Van Kleek, 1982) and to use language to talk about language (Bernstein, 1993). Children between five and eight become aware that language is an arbitrary code used to communicate with others. The development of concentration enables the child to develop the ability to focus on and process two aspects of language simultaneously, message meaning and linguistic correctness (Owens, 1988). These abilities involve an understanding of all components of the language—form, content, and use (Bernstein; Dickinson et al., 1993; Owens, 1988). Table 4.4 illustrates the metalinguistic abilities of school-age children.

TABLE 4.4 *Metalinguistic Abilities of School-Age Children*

  I. Recognizing that language is an arbitrary conventional code
      A. Understanding and using multiple-meaning words
      B. Understanding and using figurative language
      C. Using different sentence forms to express the same meaning
      D. Detecting ambiguous sentences and explaining their ambiguity

 II. Recognizing language as a system of units and rules for combining those units
      A. Segmenting words into phones and sentences into words
      B. Judging grammaticality
      C. Correcting ungrammatical sentences
      D. Applying appropriate inflections to new words

III. Recognizing that language is used for communication
      A. Judging utterances as appropriate for specific listeners or settings
      B. Awareness of the politeness of various request forms

---

Source: Bernstein, D. A. (1993). Language development: The school age years. In D. K. Bernstein & E. Tiergerman (Eds.), *Language and communication disorders in children* (3rd ed., p. 136). New York: Merrill/Macmillan.

Summary

Children enter school having developed many language skills. However, there are still many skills that develop during the school-age period. Children's syntax develops as they increase their frequency of use of compound and complex sentences. The content of language increases dramatically as their vocabulary expands and they begin to use figurative language. The function and form of language increase as children use oral language in a variety of ways. Children learn to adjust their messages to the listener and are able to repair communication breakdowns. The use of oral language in social situations increases as the peer group becomes more significant in their lives.

References and Suggested Readings

Bernstein, D. K. (1993). Language development: The school-age years. In D. K. Bernstein & E. Tiergerman (Eds.), *Language and communication disorders in children* (3rd ed., pp. 123–145). New York: Merrill.

Bjork, R. A., & Bjork, E. L. (1992). A new theory of disuse and an old theory of stimulus fluctuation. In A. F. Healy, S. M. Kosslyn, & R. M. Shiffrin (Eds.), *From learning processes to cognitive processes: Essays in honor of William K. Estes* (Vol. 2, pp. 35–67). Hillsdale, NJ: Erlbaum.

Bloom, L., & Lahey, M. (1975). *Language development and language disorders*. New York: John Wiley.

Bos, C. S., & Vaughn, S. (1998). *Strategies for teaching students with learning and behavior problems* (4th ed.). Boston: Allyn & Bacon.

Dickinson, D., Wolf, M., & Stotsky, S. (1993). Words move: The interwoven development of oral and written language. In J. B. Gleason (Ed.), *The development of language* (3rd ed., pp. 369–420). New York: Macmillan.

Dollaghan, C. (1985). Child meets word: "Fast mapping" in preschool children. *Journal of Speech and Hearing Research, 28,* 449–454.

Dollaghan, C. (1987). Fast mapping in normal and language impaired children. *Journal of Speech and Hearing Disorders, 52,* 218–222.

Evans, D. D., & Strong, C. J. (1996). What's the story? Attending, listening, telling in middle school. *Teaching Exceptional Children, 28*(3), 58–61.

Gallagher, T. M. (1991). Language and social skills: Implications for clinical assessment and intervention with school-age children. In T. M. Gallagher (Ed.), *Pragmatics of language: Clinical practice issues* (pp. 11–41). San Diego: Singular Publishing Group.

Heibeck, T., & Markman, E. (1987). Word learning in children: An examination of fast mapping. *Child Development, 58,* 1021–1034.

Kobasigawa, A. (1977). Retrieval strategies in the development of memory. In R. Kail & J. W. Hagen (Eds.), *Perspectives in the development of memory and cognition* (pp. 177–201). Hillsdale, NJ: Erlbaum.

Lahey, M. (1988). *Language disorders and language development*. Boston: Allyn & Bacon.

MacDonald, G. W., & Cornwall, A. (1995). The relationship between phonological awareness and reading and spelling achievement eleven years later. *Journal of Learning Disabilities, 28,* 523–527.

McGregor, K. K., & Leonard, L. B. (1995). Intervention for word-finding deficits in children. In M. E. Fey, J. Windsor, & S. F. Warren (Eds.), *Language intervention: Preschool through the elementary years* (pp. 85–105). Baltimore, MD: Paul H. Brookes.

Mercer, C. D. (1997). *Students with learning disabilities.* (5th ed.). Upper Saddle River, NJ: Merrill/Prentice-Hall.

Nippold, M. A. (1988). The literate lexicon. In M. A. Nippold (Ed.), *Later language development: Ages nine through nineteen* (pp. 29–47), Austin, TX: PRO-ED.

Nippold, M. A. (1992). The nature of normal and disordered word finding children and adolescents. *Topics in Language Disorders, 13*(1), 1–14.

Nippold, M. A. (1993). Adolescents' language development markers in adolescent language: Syntax, semantics and pragmatics. *Language, Speech, and Hearing Services in the Schools, 24,* 21–28.

Owens, R. E. (1988). *Language development: An introduction* (2nd ed.). Columbus, OH: Merrill.

Owens, R. E. (1995). *Language disorders: A functional approach to assessment and intervention* (2nd ed.). New York: Merrill/Macmillan.

Pease, D. M., Gleason, J. B., & Pan, B. A. (1993). Learning the meaning of words: Semantic development and beyond. In J. B. Gleason (Ed.), *The development of language* (3rd ed., pp. 116–149). New York: Macmillan.

Peck, J. (1989). Using storytelling to promote language and literacy development. *The Reading Teacher, 42,* 138–141.

Roth, F. P., & Spekman, N. J. (1986). Narrative discourse: Spontaneously generated stories of learning disabled and normally achieving students. *Journal of Speech and Hearing Disorders, 51,* 8–23.

Scott, C. M. (1995). Syntax for school age children: A discourse perspective. In M. E. Fey, J. Windsor, & S. Warren (Eds.), *Language intervention: Preschool through elementary years* (pp. 107–143). Baltimore, MD: Paul H. Brookes.

Scott, C. M., & Stokes, S. L. (1995). Measures of syntax in school age children and adolescents. *Language, Speech, and Hearing Services in the Schools, 26,* 309–319.

Smith, C. R. (1998). From gibberish to phonemic awareness: Effective decoding instruction. *Teaching Exceptional Children, 30*(6), 20–25.

Torgesen, J. K., Wagner, R. K., & Rashotte, C. A. (1994). Longitudinal studies of phonological processing and reading. *Journal of Learning Disabilities, 27,* 276–286.

Trousdale, A. M. (1990). Interactive storytelling: Scaffolding children's early narratives. *Language Arts, 67*(2), 164–173.

Van Kleek, A. (1982). The emergence of metalinguistic awareness: A cognitive framework. *Merrill Palmer Quarterly, 28,* 237–265.

Warren, A. R., & McCloskey, L. A. (1993). Pragmatics: Language in social contexts. In J. B. Gleason (Ed.), *The development of language* (3rd ed., pp. 196–237). New York: Merrill.

Wiig, E. H., & Semel, E. (1984). *Language assessment and intervention for the learning disabled* (2nd ed.). Columbus, OH: Merrill.

Windsor, J. (1995). Language impairment and social competence. In M. E. Fey, J. Windsor, & S. F. Warren (Eds.), *Language intervention: Preschool through the elementary years* (pp. 107–143). Baltimore, MD: Paul H. Brookes.

Wood, B. C. (1976). *Children and communications: Verbal and nonverbal language development.* Upper Saddle River, NJ: Prentice-Hall.

5

The Culturally and Linguistically Diverse Exceptional Learner

Martha Lue

Chapter Objectives

On completion of this chapter, the reader will be able to:

- Describe the demographic changes of culturally and linguistically diverse students in our nation's classrooms;
- Describe the federal laws implemented to ensure appropriate education provisions for culturally and linguistically diverse learners;
- Describe the role of teacher, family, and community involvement in working with diverse cultures;
- Understand the differences between language difference and language disorder, particularly as it relates to the culturally and linguistically diverse exceptional learner; and,
- Develop strategies that the classroom teacher might use in fostering a climate of cultural and linguistic acceptance of all children.

- On the last Friday of each month, Ms. Miller's class participates in a multicultural experience as part of their social studies class. This Friday, it was Mexico. The classroom was decorated in posters depicting numerous aspects of Mexico and its culture. Authentic Mexican items brought in by the teacher were part of a "show and tell" session. The biggest hit of the day was making tacos.

- At still another local elementary school, the entire student body participates in a multicultural day. The activity, coordinated by the music teacher, includes music, art, guest speakers, demonstrations, and classroom instruction. The music teacher teaches the students songs, dances, and stories about a particular culture while the classroom teacher reinforces the information and adds more in-depth information. The entire unit takes about three to four weeks. The culminating activity is a school performance by that grade for the entire student body. Parents are invited to this very special event. Finally, each student has a "passport" that they color and decorate with information on the country; they even get a stamp showing that they "visited" that country. The whole school gets involved, and all—the children, faculty, staff, and parents—have a lot of fun!

- Huerta attends a local elementary school and receives services from the self-contained programs in learning disabilities and language resource. Although he comes from a bilingual home (his parents speak almost no English at home), he is English dominant. Huerta was born in Puerto Rico, later moved to an eastern state, and finally located to his present site in a southern city. He has a history of ear infections, and is scheduled for an updated audiological evaluation. He has a repaired cleft palate, but additional cosmetic needs remain in the area of dentition. He continues to have academic and language needs and warrants specialized services for educational needs, including speaking in sentence fragments. Specific concerns are also with comprehension, problem-solving, and using language adequately in all environments.

  Recommendations include: Because Huerta has such an awareness of his language difficulties and his pragmatic skills are weak only because of serious formulating and retrieval problems, it is suggested that some arrangements be made for mainstreaming with other students so as to encourage this skill.

Scenes like the events described in *Ms. Miller's classroom* and at the other local elementary schools are taking place in schools throughout the nation as we prepare our students to learn, live, and work in the twenty-first century. In *Huerta's* case, members of the team are working collaboratively to ensure that this student is not isolated further, and that services are provided in an inclusive setting.

Demography indicates a rapidly changing composition of students in our nation's K–12 classrooms (Nissani, 1990; Correa & Tulbert, 1991; Chisholm, 1994; Parla, 1994; Green, 1997; Hodgkinson, 1998). Consider the following:

- The number of students from diverse cultures is expected to grow to 24 million, or 37 percent of the school-age population, by the year 2010;
- By the year 2000, one out of three students will be an ethnic minority (Banks & Banks, 1993);
- Currently, if students were distributed evenly across the nation's classrooms, every class of 30 students would include about 10 students from ethnic or racial minority groups. Of the 10, about 6 would be from language minority families. Two to four of these students would have limited English proficiency (LEP), of whom two would be from immigrant families. Of the 6 language minority students in the class, 4 would speak Spanish as their native language and 1 would speak an Asian language. The other language minority student would speak any one of more than a hundred languages (McLaughlin & McLeod, 1996);
- By the year 2010, the states of California, Florida, Texas, and New York will contain one-third of all United States youth. In the states of Texas and California, 57 percent of these youth will be nonwhite;
- Some culturally and linguistically diverse families may view professionals as "experts" (Chan, 1986; Correa, 1989; Cunningham, Cunningham, & O'Connell, 1986). Adding that this may also hold true for most low-income U.S. groups of any cultural affiliation, Harry (1992a) observed that "this deference may mask parents' true opinions of professional recommendations or judgements."

Challenges of Demographic Change

Bruder & Schuster (1992) observed that:

> The increasingly diverse cultures in the U.S. are perhaps this country's greatest strength. Nowhere else in the world does such a mix of people contribute to a nation's overall structure . . . But our very diversity also presents one of the most important challenges to U.S. schools today: to educate students . . . in ways that promote greater tolerance, understanding, and appreciation of the different cultures within and beyond our own "mosaic." (p. 20)

How we as a society, as a whole, and you as a classroom teacher specifically deal with these differences will, to a great extent, determine the future of the United States in the twenty-first century (Kuder, 1997). We are living and teaching in a society that is in constant change. We are teaching classes of students whose nationalities, ethnicity, race, gender, and social and economic classification may be different on a weekly basis. As a classroom teacher, you may also find that you've not received the proper amount of academic training for such a challenge.

But we all share the responsibility of providing an environment that supports and empowers individual and cultural differences. Chisholm (1994) notes that, as classroom teachers, it is our responsibility to use culturally sensitive strategies and content to ensure that all students receive equitable opportunities for academic success, personal development, and individual fulfillment.

> ### Activities
> - In your own words, define the terms *race, culture, language,* and *ethnicity.*
> - Design an activity that you might use to create better awareness of the distinct features and qualities of other languages. You may choose to use game formats, create a collage, write a children's story, or the like.

In this chapter, you will be introduced to the culture of home and school, a discussion of intercultural and intracultural competence, cultural sensitivity, and school success. A special section on issues regarding the use of Standard English will also be presented. Other discussion topics include: the role of teachers, a discussion of language difference versus language disorder, the role of the family and community involvement, provisions of services and IDEA, and some strategies that you, as a classroom teacher, might employ that would promote an atmosphere of cultural and linguistic acceptance for all students.

State and Federal Laws

Several state and federal laws have been passed that serve to promote equal educational opportunities to children of all cultural and language backgrounds, as well as to students with varying disabilities. In a previous chapter, you have already been introduced to the Education of All Handicapped Children's Act of 1975 (P.L. 94-142), and its reauthorized version, Individuals with Disabilities Education Act (IDEA, P.L. 101-476). Two additional important pieces of legislation that have had significant importance in the education of students from culturally and linguistically diverse environments are the Bilingual Education Acts of 1968 and 1976 and the court case of Lau versus Nichols (1974).

Bilingual Education Act of 1968

The Bilingual Education Act of 1968 was legislated by Congress in order to mandate schools to provide bilingual education programs. Federally funded through Title VII of the Elementary and Secondary Education Act of 1965 (PL 89-10), the Bilingual Education Act provided funds for staff and materials development as well as parent involvement for students with limited English skills (Kipp, 1999). Further, it encourages school districts to employ bilingual education practices, techniques, and methods to meet the educational needs of students who speak languages other than English. However, special assistance may vary from one district or school to another. The law was enacted for students who were defined as poor and educationally disadvantaged because of their inability to use the English language to provide them full access to the learning environment, curriculum, special services, and assessment services. It acknowledges that the educational needs of individuals with limited English proficiency cannot be met by traditional schooling in which only English is taught (Curriel, 1999).

According to the Bilingual Education Act, the terms *limited English proficiency* and *limited English proficient* refer to:

- individuals who were not born in the United States or whose native language is a language other than English;
- individuals who come from environments where a language other than English is dominant;
- individuals who are American Indian or Alaskan Natives and who come from environments where a language other than English has had a significant impact on their level of English language proficiency; and
- those who, by reason thereof, have sufficient difficulty speaking, reading, writing, or understanding the English language to deny such individuals the opportunity to learn successfully in classrooms where the language of instruction is English or to participate fully in society (20 U.S.C. 3283 (a)(1)).

Bilingual Education Act of 1976

In 1976, two years after Congress passed the Equal Educational Opportunity Act, the Chacon-Moscone Bilingual-Bicultural Education Act was established. As a result of this Act, bilingual education was mandated in the State of California, a leader in this area.

The Chacon-Moscone Act held that the lack of English language communication skills interfered in the equal educational opportunity rights of LEP (limited English proficiency) and NEP (non-English proficiency) students. Proponents of this Act declared that providing instruction and training in the student's primary languages, in addition to teaching them English (Kipp, 1999), could eliminate this interference. This legislation was further revised in 1984 and 1988 and is part of the Improving America's Schools Act of 1994 (PL 103-382) (Curriel, 1999).

Lau v. Nichols (1974). In the court case of Lau v. Nichols (1974), the father of a student named Kenny Lau asked that the child receive academic instruction in his home language, Chinese, so that the child might have an appropriate learning experience. As a result, a class action suit was then brought on behalf of 1800 Chinese students in the San Francisco Unified School District. The school district argued that the home was the institution responsible for rectifying the child's limitations in language, and that the district's responsibility was to provide equal facilities and instruction for all students. The U.S. Supreme Court held that special language programs were necessary if schools were to provide an equal educational opportunity for all students.

The Language Minority/Limited English Proficient (LEP) Child

- José, a 12-year-old sixth grader, is of Puerto Rican and Cuban descent. He and his parents are fluent in English and Spanish and speak both at home. A maternal grandmother, who speaks only Spanish, also lives with the family. His mother recalls that, as a young child, he seemed to be withdrawn at times and would become aggressive and impulsive. He also used a lot of gestures and body language. A speech-language consultation indicated that he had an articulation problem.

  When he entered kindergarten, his teacher noted that he was very delayed in vocabulary, used a lot of gestures and simple vocabulary words. Initially, she attributed this to his shyness and possible language barrier, but, as the year progressed, more articulation problems emerged. The speech-language pathologist is currently working with him on missing phonemes and improving social skills.

José represents a large portion of our nation's school-age children. Some estimates indicate that more than one-fifth of our nation's school-age children come from households in which languages other than English are spoken. It is believed that approximately two-thirds of these youngsters, described as coming from "language minority" households, themselves speak a non-English language at home (McLeod, 1996). Further,

- In public schools between 1978 and 1988, the Asian student population more than doubled and Hispanic students nearly doubled. There was a decline among both whites/non-Hispanics and blacks. No change was noted among American Indians and Alaskans (Bruder & Schuster, 1992).
- Between 1979 and 1989, the total number of children age 8 to 15 enrolled in U.S. schools who spoke a language other than English at home increased by 41 percent. Overall school enrollment at that time declined 4 percent (Bruder & Schuster, 1992).
- In 1993, virtually all students (93 percent) with limited English proficiency, including some native-born children, were enrolled in remedial language programs (Dunn, 1993).

McLeod (1997) observed that:

Many students come to school with limited English proficiency (LEP); their speaking, listening, reading, or writing skills in English are not sufficient to allow them to fully participate in traditional all-English core curriculum classes . . . Further, language minority, LEP, and immigrant youth are highly likely to be poor, to be members of ethnic or racial minority groups, and to attend segregated and poor schools.

Their families and communities may suffer stress resulting from inadequate health, social, and cultural services; low employment rates; and illegal and dangerous activities in their neighborhoods. (p. 3)

Effective Instructional Strategies: Common Attributes

Research on effective instructional strategies used with language minority/limited English proficiency (LEP) observed the following common attributes in the instructional organization of the classroom (Garcia, 1991, p. 1):

- Emphasis on functional communication between teacher and students and among fellow students;
- Organization of the instruction of basic skills and academic content around thematic units;
- Utilization of collaborative learning techniques;
- Supportive principals;
- High parental involvement.

Gersten (1996, pp. 21–22) suggests that, for teaching language minority students, effective literacy instruction should include:

- using evocative words as an explicit focus of lessons;
- using explicit strategies to help students become better readers;
- teaching children how to transfer into English what they know in their native language; and
- encouraging students to speak and write about their lives.

Culture of Home and School

Regular classrooms have their own culture. All children arrive at school with ways of speaking and interacting with adults and peers and with ideas about the purpose of schools. Oftentimes, however, the skills and strategies acquired to get along in a child's community may not be compatible with the demands of the school setting. Hence, these children may be "at risk" for becoming doubly disadvantaged:

- Their patterns of language use, behaviors, and values do not match those required in the school setting;
- Teachers, administrators, or primary caregivers fail to take advantage of the strengths that these students do possess;
- The greater the gap between the child's culture and the school's culture, the greater likelihood of failure or low pupil achievement;
- The greater the overlap between the child's culture and the school's culture, the greater the likelihood of success of high pupil achievement.

Further,

- All children bring to school the language system of their culture (Gollnick & Chinn, 1990);
- Culturally and linguistically diverse students are a heterogeneous population; gross generalizations should be avoided when learning about cultural characteristics associated with their native culture;
- Cultural language differences may create academic difficulties for some students and place them at a greater risk for special education placements (Drew, Hardman, & Logan, 1996; Morsink, Thomas, & Correa, 1991);
- Cultural differences and misinterpretations often become evident when people of different cultures attempt to communicate;
- Cultural and linguistic differences present both opportunities and challenges for teachers.

To maximize learning opportunities, it is important the teacher gain knowledge of the cultures represented in the classroom, thus allowing the opportunity to translate this knowledge into the classroom.

Activities

- Observe a real-life conversation, a movie, or interact with individuals from different cultural–linguistic backgrounds. Observe and discuss the nonverbal communication patterns, which might be different from those of your own background.
- Share and discuss your feelings regarding the issue of teaching Standard English to speakers of nonstandard dialects of English.

Intercultural/Intracultural Competence

Most culturally and linguistically diverse youngsters interact with two cultures on a daily basis: the culture of the home and the Anglo-American cultures of the schools and other social institutions. It is, then, very important that children at an early age be taught that their culture is different, not deficient, and that their culture should be acknowledged and valued.

In some Vietnamese families, for example, parents, after having moved to the United States, encourage their youngsters to master English communication, but may become concerned when, after entering school, their youngsters lose important features of their native language. Moreover, it is not uncommon for some elderly members of the family to never fully master the English language. Educators must become sensitive to these issues, fully understanding that cultural conflicts can occur when both cultures are not fully recognized.

Cultural Sensitivity and School Success

It is clearly evident that our nation is becoming increasingly more multiethnic, multicultural, and multilingual. Consider the following statistics:

- In 1985, nonwhites and Hispanics made up 29 percent of the overall elementary–secondary school population;
- In 1995, nonwhites and Hispanics increased to 34 percent of the population;
- Enrollments of Asians and Pacific Islanders are increasing more rapidly than any other group (70 percent between 1985 and 1995); Hispanics next (54 percent); African Americans (13 percent).

In the year 2000, 23 of the 25 largest public school systems were composed primarily of minority students. Research further suggests that in the twenty-first century, between 25 percent and 38 percent of school-age children will be culturally and linguistically diverse from the current majority Anglo-American population.

Communication Style and Culture

Differences in rules governing eye contact, physical space between speakers, use of gestures and facial expression, and use of silence need to be considered (Fad, 1995; Heward, 2000). Cultural clashes may occur when people in authority are not able to recognize or acknowledge that other cultures or languages of students are indeed legitimate (Keulen, Weddington, & DeBose, 1998).

Effective Home and School Collaboration

For children to be successful in school, effective collaboration between home and school must occur at all levels. For some families, the school is not viewed as "user-friendly." In contrast, some Caucasian teachers may feel that African-American parents may be apathetic and uninterested in their children's educational and social-emotional development. This points out a need for sensitivity to cultural and linguistic differences by all.

Research suggests that teachers' attitudes and expectations toward particular groups will affect their behavior toward these groups and may also influence students' performance. Morsink, Thomas, and Correa (1991) suggest that understanding the acculturation process of families from various ethnic groups is a necessary prerequisite to working effectively with them. Questions to be asked by the professional include:

- How many years has the family been in the United States?
- What were the family's living conditions in their native country?
- Is the family literate in their native language?

- Does the family have respect for elders and people in authority?
- Do extended family members play a role in the family system?

Further research done by Cazden, John, and Hymes (1972) indicated the importance of the teacher's understanding of linguistic differences as a vehicle for enabling teachers to "hear through" children's language and to listen for their meanings rather than their errors. Culturally sensitive educators provide opportunities throughout the school day that support the child's learning style.

Language Difference versus Language Disorder

Ours is a society made up of many cultures and languages. Each of us uses language differently. Hedge (1995) noted: "[I]n order to understand a language, its use, its diversity, and its disorders, it is necessary to understand the broader context of that language" (p. 415). Therefore, it is helpful at this time to review some important considerations in the discussion of language (ASHA, 1982, p. 949):

- language evolves within specific historical, social, and cultural contexts;
- language is rule-governed;
- language learning and use are determined by the interaction of biological, cognitive, psychological, and environmental factors; and
- effective use of language for communication requires a broad understanding of human interactions, including such associated factors as nonverbal cues, motivation, and sociocultural roles.

How, then, can you, as a classroom teacher, determine when a child's language usage is different or if it is disordered? A language difference, in and of itself, may not require intervention and remediation (Thomas & Carmack, 1990). However, those students in your classroom who are found to be language disordered by a team of professionals will require intervention and remediation. Thomas and Carmack define language as being disordered when "it interferes with communication, calls unfavorable attention to itself, or causes its user to be maladjusted" (p. 18).

If you are unsure about whether a child has a speech or language problem, you are encouraged to refer the child for testing by a speech, language, or hearing professional. Speech-language pathologists are specially trained to serve as consultants to teachers and other professionals on dialectal variations and modifications.

Language Differences and the Issue of Standard English

Some of the youngsters in your classroom will enter speaking differently than other children with whom you may have had some experience. For the majority of these youngsters, there may not be anything "wrong" with their speech and they will not require any special educational services. Dialect speakers may face significant barriers as they enter and progress through the school (Bountress, 1994). The speech-language pathologist will be instrumental in developing strategies that may assist the student.

For still another group of students, many of whom may be of African-American descent, their language use may not be the "standard" that is usually heard in most middle-class families. Thus, the issue of Standard English should be addressed. The population that speaks another language or dialect outside of Standard English has increased dramatically. As a classroom teacher, it is important that you are able to differentiate between typical and atypical phonological development in children who do not speak Standard American English.

The question arises—Should Standard English be taught? What are the benefits? Research suggests that teaching Standard English to culturally and linguistically diverse students is important because these students may be at risk for academic failure. Sometimes, however, teachers whose only language is English may feel unqualified to teach non-English speakers. Further, offering instruction "to improve" speech may send the mixed message of criticism not only of the language but also of the person. Several approaches to understanding this sensitive and complex issue have been reported:

Robbins (1989) described a unit of study designed to emphasize "Broadcast English" as a register to be used in certain situations (e.g., job interviews, reporting, and presenting in class). Instruction in voice and diction was given to the members in the group. Results indicated that the students involved not only began to speak Standard English in certain situations, but that much of their nonstandard dialect could be neutralized when it was advantageous to conform to someone else's expectations. Journal writing is also an effective tool, because students write on any topic they choose. Teachers, in turn, read the journal entries and respond.

The classroom teacher may also try using reading materials that deal with the culture of the student. It is highly likely that bicultural readers comprehend and remember materials that deal with their own culture better than those of another culture.

Family and Community Involvement

A school that affirms cultural responsiveness will make an effort to integrate the community in its total program, suggest Gollnick and Chin (1990). Effective family/community and school programs are based on planning that emphasizes parent (family) involvement to help children toward better achievement and adjustment in school.

While parents may have high academic expectations for their children, they may not perceive a particular school as user-friendly. The following strategies may be helpful in fostering greater understanding:

- Use teacher aides or assistants who are proficient in the family's native language or culture;
- Use language that parents can understand and use that language sensitively in the family's community;

- Provide a home visitor. Schools must reach out to families and homes and in neighborhoods to provide information, materials, and guidance to that large constituency that does not come to school;
- Get to know the parents' strength and culture. Build on the strength by having parents come to class to lead special projects or discussions;
- Use schools to connect students and families with community resources that provide educational enrichment and support.

Provision of Services and the Individuals with Disabilities Education Act (IDEA)

While all children with special needs are entitled to a free, appropriate education, as mandated by the Individuals with Disabilities Education Act, it is becoming increasingly clear that there are factors that serve to complicate the provision of appropriate services for students of color. These factors, as delineated by Smith, Finn, and Dowdy (1993) include lack of:

- trained personnel who can test children in their native language, and who are able to interpret performances that adequately describe children's linguistic and cultural characteristics;
- adequate assessment instruments and procedures for identifying handicapping conditions among culturally diverse individuals;
- instructional materials for culturally and linguistically diverse individuals;
- necessary training and expertise needed to implement effective bilingual special education programs.

The Preservice Educator and Cultural Responsiveness

There continues to be growing concern about the disparity of minority students and minority teachers in our nation's classrooms. Further, few students in teacher education programs come from urban areas, and only 15 percent of students express interest in teaching in an urban area.

Further, Coballes-Vega (1982) observes that the majority of prospective teachers are white females, a situation that stands in sharp contrast to the backgrounds of the students they will teach. Glenn (1989) notes, however, that simply adopting new requirements or issuing new instructions to teachers does not automatically lead to more effective teaching for culturally diverse students.

The goal of any teacher education program should be to guide the systematic transmission of knowledge and information regarding culturally different and linguistically different learners, to encourage the internalization of behavior and/or attitude consistent with the knowledge learned, and to reinforce the desire to know/learn about cultures and languages different from those of the prospective teacher's own.

Strategies for Instructing Diverse Populations: The Role of Teachers

For children, teachers are viewed as models of appropriate or expected behavior. The teacher, directly or indirectly, controls much of the activity in the learning setting and is responsible for all that occurs for the children during the day. To successfully work with children of various cultural, linguistic, or ethnic backgrounds, the teacher must have a positive attitude about cultural sensitivity.

Cultural sensitivity, add Banks and Banks (1993), involves not only what a teacher does, but what a teacher says. The teacher must be sensitive to his or her own racial attitudes, behaviors, and the statements that are made about ethnic groups in the classroom. For example, in role-playing about Black History, children other than children of color may be encouraged to play roles of Native Americans or African-American individuals. Children of color may, likewise, take the role of Caucasians or people of other groups.

Understanding One's Own Culture

In order for one to understand another's culture, it is imperative that one understands his or her own beliefs, values, and cultural history. Exercises in cultural awareness are cited in several references (Garcia & Ortiz, 1988; Slade & Conoley, 1989; Randall-David, 1989).

Storytelling

Storytelling is an activity that can assist children and preservice educators in acknowledging others' cultures. The art of storytelling, noted Zabel (1991), predates any other form of oral history. Storytelling in the past has been used to instruct, to illustrate, and to guide the thinking of students. In addition, storytelling can be an excellent vehicle by which to share another's culture. The book, *Mufaro's Beautiful Daughters*, by John Steptoe (1987), can be used to assist students in sharing, understanding, and appreciating another's culture.

Books

While some books may discuss culturally and linguistically diverse youngsters in a negative sense, it becomes your role as teacher to ensure that presentations of the material be done in a culturally sensitive manner. Activities that capitalize on the power of literature to promote intercultural and multicultural appreciation can be presented in an effort to promote cultural awareness and sensitivity. With special needs children, further adaptations may be required, based on the learning style and exceptionality of the student.

Helping the Culturally Diverse Student Become an Active Member in the Classroom

Whether it is due to language, clothes, or customs, some students from the majority culture may view students from cultures other then their own as truly different and may limit their interactions with them (Salend, 1998). Strategies must be developed that will ensure that all students become active participants in the learning environment.

Wagner (1981) offers five suggestions for ways teachers can develop positive attitudes and behaviors toward culturally diverse students:

1. Become knowledgeable about the culturally different student. The teacher should take the time to get to know more about the student's background by reading, interviewing, observing, and visiting. If the teacher does not do this, he or she will not understand why the child has trouble adjusting in the classroom. Learning about the student's vocabulary and interests will help the teacher have an open mind about cultural differences; visit the student's neighborhood and also visit the parents in order to understand "where the child is coming from." Dr. Jaqueline Irvine, the Charles Howard Candler Professor of Urban Education at Emory University, sums it up this way (1999):

> Culture can be learned. Take a white teacher from Montgomery County, Maryland who goes to Argentina. What do they do? They read about Argentina, they study, they make trips to Argentina. They talk to people from Argentina. Teachers need to adopt the same spirit of learning that they adopt when they go to Europe, to Argentina, while they learn the cultures of other children. . . . (p. 32)

2. Avoid stereotyping or being biased; become accepting. The teacher should emphasize the likenesses of his or her culture and the student's culture instead of placing too much emphasis on differences. It is easier to adjust to a culturally different classroom with the help of an unbiased teacher. It is important for the teacher not to prejudge or have preconceived ideas about the student's culture.

3. Accept each student as an individual. The teacher should not assume that all students from a given cultural group are alike. These students may need more individual attention and the teacher has to take the time to carefully praise and correct mistakes.

4. Enhance the student's self-concept. Help the student become secure as part of the group while retaining his or her cultural identity. The teacher should work at creating a culturally sensitive environment.

5. Be one's self. The students can detect a phony; the teacher needs to be honest with him- or herself about whether or not he or she is comfortable in a setting. The teacher must also be a model for the class and accept all students regardless of race, color, or background.

Acculturation

Multicultural bilingual educators have registered concern with the lack of attention given to the acculturation process in which many children from culturally/ linguistically diverse populations find themselves as they leave home to attend school. Questions presented here suggest one model of obtaining specific linguistic and sociocultural information on which decisions are made regarding instructional materials and strategies (Barrera, 1994):

- Is a language other than English spoken in the home? If yes, to what degree and by whom? What is the child's degree of involvement with that language— receptively and/or expressively?
- Would you and your families consider yourselves culturally diverse? In what ways? Would you identify with a particular ethnic group?
- What aspects of your family life would you consider unique or special?
- How long have you lived in this area? Where have you lived before you came to this area?
- Besides parents and siblings, who are some of the people that you might consider family? If the family's response to these questions indicates significant cultural/linguistic diversity, home visits may be advisable to obtain more information.

Strategies for Developing a Culturally Responsive Classroom

The classroom environment is one of the best ways to begin developing a culturally responsive perspective that values and accepts all cultures. Students are generally responsive to learning about each other's cultural attitudes and values that are different from their own. The following general ideas can assist the teacher in implementing this very important task:

- Check to see if your school has reference books available with a list of people that you can get to come to your school or individual classrooms. Utilize speakers that can complement and reinforce subjects you may be teaching in your class.
- For this strategy, you'll need the book, *The Greatest of All: A Japanese Folktale,* retold by Eric A. Kimmell, illustrated by Giora Carmi, and published by Holiday House. The haiku at the end of the story addresses lessons of modesty and patience. Encourage students to write their own haiku. Have them copy their poems onto white or gray paper that has been cut in the shape of small boulders. Post the poems on a bulletin board.
- As a teacher, it is your responsibility to serve as a model for tolerance and acceptance. You may wish to review articles from various educational magazines

such as *Creative Classrooms* and *Instructor* that deal with various aspects of discrimination, prejudice, and stereotyping.

- During Hispanic Awareness month, a local middle school decorated an entire hallway with maps and other information pertaining to Hispanic Awareness. This allowed other students the exposure to the display every day on their way to lunch. The school also sponsored a trivia contest. Questions were read as a part of the morning announcements, and prizes were awarded to students who got questions correct. Poster contests can be included that involve research from the library.

- Obtain a copy of Crystal Kuyendall's book, *From Rage to Hope: Reclaiming Black and Hispanic Youth* (1992), National Educational Services, 1610 W. Third Street, P. O. Box 8, Bloomington, IN 47402. This book radiates hope. In it, the teacher can demonstrate hope by making eye contact in a direct, sincere, loving, and encouraging way by commenting privately on specific behavior, and expecting the best from each student.

Summary

Ours is a nation comprised of people from different backgrounds, experiences, ethnic and cultural groups, and expectations. Demography indicates a rapidly changing composition in our nation's classrooms as we begin the twenty-first century.

How we as a society embrace these differences will indeed have a tremendous impact on the lives of each of us. It then becomes our responsibility as teachers to provide academic, social, and emotional support that empowers individual cultural and language differences.

This chapter has attempted to present the reader with some strategies that classroom teachers might employ that will promote an atmosphere of acceptance for all learners. A historical perspective that revisited some state and federal laws that led to provisions for cultural and linguistic diverse learners was presented. The role of the teacher and the importance of community and family involvement were explored. An understanding of language difference versus language disorder was examined.

Finally, keep in mind that the classroom teacher, in collaboration with the child's parents, can have a major impact on the child's communicative development and skills. This is true for all children, but especially those whose first language is not English. Teachers' cultural sensitivity and acceptance of all cultures and all children is vital for the success of all students.

References and Suggested Readings

Adger, C. T., Wolfram, W., and Detwyler, J. (1993). Language differences. *TEACHING Exceptional Children, 26,* 44–47.

American Association of Colleges for Teacher Education (1990). *The next level: Minority teacher supply and demand: A policy statement.*

ERIC Document Reproduction Service No. ED 332 980.

American Speech-Language-Hearing Association. (1982). Definitions: Communication disorders and variations, *ASHA, 24,* 949–950.

Banks, J. A., & Banks, C. A. (Eds.). (1993). *Multicultural education: Issues and perspectives* (2nd ed.). Boston: Allyn & Bacon.

Barrera, I. (1994). Effective and appropriate instruction for all children: The challenge of cultural/linguistic diversity and young children with special needs. *Topics in Early Childhood Special Education, 13*(4), 461–485.

Bountress, N. G. (1994). The classroom teacher and the language different student: Why, when, and how of intervention. *Preventing School Failure, 38*(4), 10–15.

Bruder, I., & Schuster, J. (1992, October). Multicultural education: Responding to the demographics of change. *Electronic Learning, 12*(2), 20–27.

Cazden, C., John, V., & Hymes, P. (Eds.). (1972). *Functions of language in the classroom.* New York: Teachers College Press.

Chan, S. (1986). Parents of exceptional Asian children. In M. K. Vitano and P. C. Chinn (Eds.), *Exceptional Asian children and youth* (pp. 36–53). Reston, VA: Council for Exceptional Children.

Cheng, L. (1998). *Intervention strategies for CLD students with speech-language disorders. Compendium: Writing on effective practices for culturally and linguistically diverse exceptional learners.* Reston, VA: Council for Exceptional Children.

Chisholm, I. M. (1994, Winter). Preparing teachers for multicultural classrooms. *Journal of Educational Issues of Language Minority Students, 14,* 43–68.

Coballes-Vega, C. (1982). Considerations in teaching culturally diverse children. *ERIC Clearinghouse on Teacher Education.* ERIC Document #: EDO-SP-90-2: Washington, DC.

Cole, P. A., & Taylor, O. L. (1990). Performance of working-class African-American children on three tests of articulation. *Language, Speech and Hearing Services in Schools, 21,* 171–176.

Collison, M. (1999). Preparing teachers for urban classrooms. *Black Issues in Higher Education, 16*(20), 31–32.

Correa, V. I. (1989). Involving culturally diverse families in the educational process. In S. H. Fradd and M. S. Wiesmantel (Eds.), *Meeting the needs of culturally and linguistically diverse students: A handbook for educators* (pp. 138–144). Boston: College Hill.

Correa, V. I., & Tulbert, B. (1991). Teaching culturally diverse students. *Preventing School Failure, 35*(3), 20–25.

Covert, B., & Gorski, P. (1998, June 24). The multicultural niche: A working definition. Initial thoughts on multicultural education. *Multicultural Pavilion.* Available on line: http://curry.edschool.virginia.edu/go/multicultural/initial.html

Cummins, J. (1986). Empowering minority students: A framework for intervention. *Harvard Educational Review, 56,* 18–35.

Cunningham, K., Cunningham, K. L., & O'Connell, J. C. (1986). Impact of differing cultural perceptions on special education service delivery. *Rural Special Education Quarterly, 8*(1), 2–8.

Curriel, F. (1999). Bilingual education. In S. L. Zepeda & M. Langenbach (Eds), *Special programs in regular schools: Historical foundations, standards, and contemporary issues* (pp. 15–27). Boston: Allyn & Bacon.

Drew, C., Hardman, M., & Logan, D. (1996). *Mental retardation: A life cycle approach* (6th ed.). New York: Merrill/Prentice-Hall.

Dunn, R. (1997). The goals and track record of multicultural education. *Educational Leadership, 54,* 74.

Dunn, W. (1993). Educating diversity. *American Demographics,* 38–43.

Fad, K. (1995). Communication disorders. In T. Smith, E. Polloway, J. Patton, and C. Dowdy (Eds.), *Teaching students with special needs in inclusive settings* (pp. 248–285). Boston: Allyn & Bacon.

Garcia, E. (1988). *Effective schooling for language minority students* (New Focus No. 1). Washington, DC: National Clearinghouse for Bilingual Education.

Garcia, E. (1991). *Education of linguistically and culturally diverse students: Effective instructional practices. Educational practice report number 1.* Santa Cruz, CA, and Washington, DC: National Center for Research on Cultural Diversity and Second Language Learning. (ERIC Document Reproduction Service No. ED 338 099)

Garcia, S., & Ortiz, A. B. (1988, June). Preventing inappropriate referrals of language minority students to special education (New Focus 5). Washington, DC: National Clearinghouse for Bilingual Education.

Gay, G. (1993). Building cultural bridges: A bold proposal for teacher education. *Education and Urban Society, 25*(3), 284–299.

Gersten, R. C. (1996). The double demands of teaching English language learners. *Educational Leadership, 53*(5), 18–22.

Gersten, R., and Woodward, J. (1994). The language minority student and special education: Issues, trends, and paradoxes. *Exceptional Children, 60,* 310–322.

Glenn, C. L. (1989). Just schools for minority children. *Phi Delta Kappan, 70*(10), 772–776.

Gollnick, D., & Chinn, P. (1990). *Multicultural education in a pluralistic society* (3rd ed.). Columbus, OH: Merrill.

Green, E. J. (1997). Guidelines for serving linguistically and culturally diverse young children. *Early Childhood Education Journal, 24*(3), 147–154.

Harris, K. C. (1991). An expanded view on consultation competencies for educators serving culturally and linguistically diverse exceptional students. *Teacher Education and Special Education, 14*(1), 25–29.

Harry, B. (1992a). *Cultural diversity, families, and the special education system: Communication and empowerment.* New York: Teachers College Press.

Harry, B. (1992b). Developing cultural self-awareness: The first step in value clarification for early interventionists. *Topics in Early Childhood Special Education, 12*(3), 333–350.

Hawley, C. (1997, June 29). Ideas for working with students who speak English as a second language. *Teacher Talk, 2*(2) [On line]. Available: http://education.indiana.edu/cas/tt/v2i2/ideas.html

Hedge, M. N. (1995). *Introduction to communication disorders.* Austin, TX: PRO-ED.

Heward, W. L. (2000). *Exceptional children* (6th ed.). Upper Saddle River, NJ: Merrill/Prentice-Hall.

Hodgkinson, H. L. (1985). *All One System: Demographics of Education—Kindergarten through Graduate School.* Washington, DC: Institute for Educational Leadership.

Hodgkinson, H. L. (1998). Speech presented at the Faculty Center for Teaching and Learning, University of Central Florida, Orlando, FL.

Ingrassia, M., and Rossi, M. (1994, February). The limits of tolerance? *Newsweek,* p. 47.

Jones, E., and Derman-Sparks, L. (1992). Meeting the challenge of diversity. *Young Children, 47*(2), 12–18.

Keulen, J. E., Weddington, G. T. & DeBose, C. E. (1998). *Speech, language, learning, and the African American Child.* Boston: Allyn & Bacon.

Kipp, P. (1999). Bilingual Education Act. [On line]. Available: http://www.gseis.ucla.edu/courses/ed191/assignment1/kipp.html

Kuder, S. J. (1997). *Teaching students with language and communication disabilities.* Boston: Allyn & Bacon.

Lau v. Nichols, 411 U.S. 563 (1974).

Lucas, T., Henze, R., & Donato, R. (1990). Promoting the success of Latino language minority students: An exploratory study of six high schools. *Harvard Educational Review, 60,* 315–339.

Martin, P., & Midgley, E. (1994). Immigration to the United States: Journey to an uncertain destination. *Population Bulletin, 49*(2), 2–47.

McLaughlin, B., & McLeod, B. (1996). Educating all our students: Improving education for children from culturally and linguistically diverse backgrounds. *Final Report of the National Center for Research on Cultural Diversity and Second Language Learning, 1* (June). University of California, Santa Cruz.

McLeod, B. (1996). School reform and student diversity: Exemplary schooling for language minority students. *NCBE Resource Collection Series,* 1–37.

McLoyd, V. C. (1990). Minority children: Introduction to the special issue. *Child Development, 61,* 263–266.

Moll, L. (1988). Educating Latino students. *Language Arts, 64,* 315–324.

Morsink, C. V., Thomas, C. C., and Correa, V. I. (1991). *Interactive teaming: Consultation and collaboration in special programs.* New York: Merrill.

Moyers, S. (1993, January). Bridging the culture gap. *Instructor,* 31–33.

National Association for the Education of Young Children. (1989). *Code of Ethics,* Washington, DC: Author.

Nissani, H. (1990). Early childhood programs for language minority children (*FOCUS: Occasional Papers in Bilingual Education, 2*). Washington, DC: National Clearinghouse for Bilingual Education.

Olmsted, P. P. (1992). Where did our diversity come from? *High Scope Resource, 11*(3), 4–9.

One America: The Face of America. The President's Initiative on Race. [On line]. Available: http://www/whitehouse.gov/Initiatives/OneAmerica/face.html

Oyer, H. J., Crowe, B., and Haas, W. H. (1994). *Speech, language, and hearing disorders: A guide for the teacher* (2nd ed.). Boston: Allyn & Bacon.

Parla, S. (1994, Summer). Educating teachers for cultural and linguistic diversity: A model for all teachers. *New York State Association for Bilingual Education Journal, 9,* 16.

Preparing teachers for urban classrooms (1999, November 25). *Black Issues in the Higher Education, 16*(20), 31–32.

Randall-David, E. (1989). *Strategies for working with culturally diverse communities and clients.* Washington, DC: Association for the Care of Children's Health.

Robbins, J. F. (1989). 'Broadcast English' for nonstandard dialect speakers. *Education Digest, 54,* 52–53.

Rounds, K. A., Weil, M., and Bishop, K. K. (1994). Practice with culturally diverse families of young children with disabilities. *Families in Society, 75,* 3–15.

Salend, S. (1998). *Effective mainstreaming: Creating inclusive classrooms* (3rd ed.). Upper Saddle River, NJ: Merrill.

Slade, J., & Conoley, C. (1989). Multicultural experiences for the special educator. *Teaching Exceptional Children, 22*(1).

Sleeter, C. E. (1992). Restructuring schools for multicultural education. *Journal of Teacher Education, 43,* 141–148.

Smith, T. E. C., Finn, D. M., & Dowdy, C. A. (1993). *Teaching students with mild disabilities.* Orlando, FL: Harcourt Brace Jovanovich.

Steptoe, J. (1987). *Mufaro's beautiful daughters: An African tale.* New York: Lothrop.

Thomas, P., & Carmack, F. (1990). *Speech and language: detecting and correcting special needs.* Boston: Allyn & Bacon.

Tiedt, P. L., & Tiedt, I. M. (1999). *Multicultural teaching: A handbook of activities, information, and resources* (5th ed.). Boston: Allyn &Bacon.

Wagner, H. (1981). Working with the culturally different student. *Education, 101*(4), 353–358.

Williams, B. F. (1992). Changing demographics: Challenges for educators. *Intervention in Schools and Community, 27*(3), 157–163.

Yates, J. R., and Ortiz, A. A. (1991). Professional development needs of teachers who serve exceptional language minorities in today's schools. *Teacher Education and Special Education, 14,* 11–18.

Zabel, M. K. (1991). Storytelling, myths, and folktales: Strategies for multicultural inclusion. *Preventing School Failure, 36*(1), 32–34.

6

Teaching Language Skills to Students with Mild Disabilities

Mary Little

Chapter Objectives

After reading this chapter, the reader will be able to discuss:

- Some of the considerations when developing and implementing language programs for students with mild disabilities;
- Other considerations that must be taken into account for instruction, specific competencies to be mastered, and instructional approaches used in providing language strategies for students with mild disabilities; and
- Specific information about students with disabilities that may impact language development.

- Samantha is nineteen and currently taking three regular education classes in the local high school. When she was born, the diagnosis was Down syndrome with little potential for a successful adult life. Samantha's mother accepted the medical diagnosis but rejected the prognosis that she would not learn enough to be self-sufficient as an adult.

  Samantha's mother was not pleased with the early intervention programs so she returned to college to prepare to teach students with mental handicaps. She consistently opposed the limited time allocation for speech therapy indicated on the IEP and insisted that her daughter would be successful in the mildly handicapped class. Although the therapy time was increased, she continued her speech classes in the private clinic. She was convinced that the language delay shadowed her daughter's intellectual potential.

When the first reevaluation in the elementary school was completed, the psychologist explained to her mother that, although Samantha's intellectual quotient was 76, she would not be placed in a regular classroom, but in the mildly handicapped class, because her adaptive behaviors were below her age level. Still defiant, yet realizing that her daughter's expressive skills in written and oral language were not at the level of her receptive and processing skills, she continued to provide tutoring support throughout the elementary years. For three years, Samantha has been in regular high school classes. She expects to graduate with a regular diploma within two years.

Acquisition and mastery of language synthesizes complex and multifaceted components that must be skillfully interwoven within social settings. Speech, language, and communication skills are developed through direct and indirect interactions within all of our social settings. Articulation of the sounds, precise vocabulary, speech, pitch, and nonverbal gestures are only a few of the isolated skills that merge when a message is communicated through the interaction of a speaker and listener.

The previous chapters have set the stage for this chapter:

- the vocabulary established the script for this production of language acquisition through our teaching;
- the story of the development of language skills provided the background and foreshadowing of the plot;
- some of the characters have been introduced—those being some of the children with language disorders and disabilities.

This chapter will further define the considerations when developing and implementing programs for language acquisition by children with mild disabilities within the schools: instruction, specific competencies to be mastered, instructional approaches, and example lessons will be shared in discreet format.

Also, specific information about students with disabilities, such as *Samantha*, that may impact language development will be discussed. However, the challenge is to remember that language acquisition is a social, interactive process that relies on a multitude of mastered skills that continuously develop.

BOX 6.1 • *Considerations for All Students with Disabilities*

- Multidisciplinary team should employ a goal-oriented approach for development of the Individual Education Plan (IEP) based on the assessed needs and the anticipated outcomes for each individual student.
- There should be collaboration among speech-language pathologist, special and general education teachers, parents, administrators, student, and other service providers for planning, implementation, and continuous progress monitoring.
- Implementation of research-based instructional programs, curricular materials, methods, and various cognitive and metacognitive strategies to assure attainment of goals and objectives as stated.
- Individualized instruction with various accommodations and modifications, as needed by each individual student.
- Maximized instruction of stated goals and objectives across all settings, including classrooms, home, lunchrooms, etc.
- Continuous monitoring of and communication of established goals among team members.

Students with Mental Retardation

The existence of mental retardation usually is identified early in a young child's life, due to the developmental delay evidenced with the child's overall functioning in gross and fine motor skills, and usually confirmed with intellectual and behavioral assessments. Mental retardation has been defined as intellectual functioning that is significantly below average, observed during the developmental years, and accompanied by deficits in adaptive behavior. The regulations for the Individuals with Disabilities Education Act (IDEA) provide the following technical definition for mental retardation:

> Mental retardation means significantly subaverage general intellectual functioning existing concurrently with deficits in adaptive behavior and manifested during the developmental period that adversely affects a child's educational performance.

In explaining the definition of mental retardation, Drew, Hardman, and Logan (1996) add that the phrase, *significantly subaverage intellectual functioning*, is used to define an IQ standard score of approximately 70 to 75 or below. This IQ score must be based on assessment from individually administered general intelligence tests that were developed for the specific purpose of assessing intellectual functioning.

Recent statistics report that 2 percent to 3 percent of the general population is people with mental retardation. According to data reported to the U.S. Department of Education by states, in the 1997–1998 school year, over 600,000 students ages six to twenty-one were classified as having mental retardation. This figure, however, does not include students with more severe mental retardation or multiple handicaps.

Due to the range of severity of cognitive abilities within the category of mental retardation, associated language deficits and disabilities can range from developmental delays commensurate with intellectual functioning to the inability to communicate the most basic needs. Depending on the extent of the impairment—mild, moderate, severe, or profound—individuals with mental retardation will develop differently in academic, social, and vocational skills. Communication may be through the most basic nonverbal techniques or with the use of symbol boards and augmentative and assistive communication systems. When speech is intelligible, it may be socially inappropriate or inadequate. Delay in the language skills may be reflected in all areas of academics. For example, reading achievement across the academic subjects and vocational training will be affected if vocabulary development has been delayed. Students with mental retardation can have associated speech problems in the area of articulation, but not as an identifying characteristic of this disability.

Activity

Before continuing with this chapter, can you describe the differences among the components of language: speech, language, and communication? (HINT: Review Chapter 1, if uncertain.)

Students with mental retardation may follow the developmental sequence of language acquisition, use, and comprehension, but they will not progress at the same rate of intellectual functioning. Therefore, the extent and rate of acquisition of their total development of language will not be that for "typical" learners. Therefore, it is critical to clearly delineate the needed language and communication goals for the individual student considering his or her long-term life outcomes through the Individualized Education Planning (IEP) process. It is also very important to consider developmentally appropriate programming. That is, if an eighteen-year-old student with mental retardation is learning functional vocabulary words (e.g., *stop, yield, go,* etc.), the words should be associated with learning to drive or work, not a primer reader with pictures.

Activity

Identify the components of language discussed in the first chapter. Create a graphic organizer and mnemonic to remember several characteristics of each of the components.

BOX 6.2 • *Considerations for Students with Mental Retardation***

- Build on existing communication systems and skills of students through observations of current communication strategies. Observe across settings, routines, and activities.
- Create a classroom climate of trust and respect, with opportunities for language stimulation and development.
- Select functional communication goals and identify powerful teaching opportunities by deciding if the communication behavior will enhance independence of the student.
- Instruct within authentic settings, using concrete examples, with intrinsically reinforcing activities. Build on the desire to communicate with and interact with specific people and life activities that are motivating (lunchroom, interacting with peers, etc.).
- Facilitate the maximum use and reinforcement of the new language and communication skills. Collaborate with other team members, educators, family members, and peers that will assist this process.
- Determine reinforcement and monitoring of the new communication and language skills.
- Ensure the maintenance and generalization of the new behavior through consistent monitoring across various settings.

**Activities synthesized from Ostrosky, Drasgow, & Halle, 1999; Oyer, Hall, & Haas, 1994; Thomas & Carmack, 1990.

Students with Learning Disabilities

The federal definition of *learning disabilities* is "a disorder in one or more of the basic psychological processes involved in understanding or in using spoken or written language, which may manifest itself in the areas of listening, thinking, writing, reading, spelling, or computing mathematics" (IDEA, 1997). Learning disabilities include such conditions as perceptual disabilities, minimal brain dysfunction, dyslexia, and developmental aphasia, but are not a primary result of visual, hearing, or motor disabilities, mental retardation, or environmental, cultural, or economic causes. Although definitions of learning disabilities vary among the states, the Interagency Committee on Learning Disabilities concluded that 5 percent to 10 percent is a reasonable estimate of students with learning disabilities in schools.

Students with learning disabilities may exhibit a combination of characteristics that may mildly, moderately, or severely impair the learning process. Learning disabilities are characterized by a significant difference in the child's achievement in some areas, as compared to the overall intelligence. Academically, students with learning disabilities may exhibit a wide range of traits, including problems with language as evidenced in reading comprehension, spoken language, written language, and reasoning abilities. Receptive and expressive language, in both the written and oral forms, can be a significant area for remediation. Difficulties will be evidenced in reading, writing, spelling, and comprehending oral and written directions across each of the academic settings. The discrepancies between expectations and achievement for the students with learning disabilities increase without intense remediation in these areas.

In addition, associated neurological characteristics of learning disabilities include difficulties with perceptual coordination, impulsivity, hyperactivity, and motor and organizational disorders. Communication within social settings can be affected as pragmatics depend on the ability to use appropriate nonverbal skills within a social context. Students with learning disabilities can be socially excluded due to poor communication and language skills. This can result in additional frustrations and decreased self-esteem. Because learning disabilities are manifested in a variety of academic and associated behavioral patterns, the educational implications are best again discussed with close collaboration among special education teachers, speech and language clinicians (as appropriate), parents, the student, administrators, and general education teachers. This team approach is important for educating the student with learning disabilities, beginning with the assessment process and continuing through the development and monitoring of the Individual Education Program (IEP). Instruction should capitalize on the student's strengths, while providing clear goals, high expectations, and cognitive and metacognitive strategies to develop the necessary language skills. Research clearly suggests that explicit and direct instruction of specific skills to mastery by the individual student produces the greatest achievement levels (Carnine, 1990; Torgesen, 1996). Use of technology (word processing computer programs with spelling and grammar assists, calculators, etc.) can help students with learning disabilities in particular areas.

Activity

Listen to lectures in your classes. Identify any language cueing techniques or strategies used by the speaker.

Students with Serious Emotional Disturbances

As the exact numbers of students with learning disabilities are difficult to accurately establish, so, too, are the terms and defining characteristics as elusive when identifying students who have been described with emotional, behavioral, or mental disorders. Serious emotional disturbances (SED) are defined as follows:

A condition exhibiting one or more of the following characteristics over a long period of time and to a marked degree that adversely affects educational performance:

BOX 6.3 • *Considerations for Students with Learning Disabilities***

- Once instructional goals and objectives have been established, teach metacognitive strategies to assist memory, organization of materials, and recall. For example, explicitly teach similarities with common sounds.
- Instruct using various modalities to assure mastery of instructional objectives. Write, read, pronounce, draw, and visually organize the new information across various settings and using various modalities.
- Relate new information to prior learning and stated lesson objectives, and provide rationale for the language lesson.
- Teach to mastery of the objective or goal. Provide maximum opportunities to practice the new skills, providing corrective feedback. Teach for automaticity.
- Provide the explicit connections for students, e.g., the reading vocabulary words and weekly spelling words that all have the same initial sounds, etc.
- Provide research-based instruction of methods, materials, and strategies that have validated effectiveness.
- Facilitate the maximum use and reinforcement of the new language and communication skills. Collaborate with other team members, educators, family members, and peers that will assist this process. Incorporate cooperative learning structures into instruction.
- Determine reinforcement and monitoring of the new communication and language skills.
- Ensure the maintenance and generalization of the new behavior through consistent monitoring across various settings.

**Activities synthesized from Brinton & Fujiki, 1998; Deshler & Schumaker, 1987; Frost & Emery, 1995; Mercer & Mercer, 1999; Oyer, Hall, & Haas, 1994; Shaywitz, 1996; Thomas & Carmack, 1990.

- An inability to learn that cannot be explained by intellectual, sensory, or health factors;
- An inability to build or maintain satisfactory interpersonal relationships with peers or teachers;
- Inappropriate types of behavior or feelings under normal circumstances;
- A general pervasive mood of unhappiness or depression; or
- A tendency to develop physical symptoms or fears associated with personal or school problems [Code of Federal Regulations, Title 34, 300.7(b)(9)].

The causes of serious emotional disturbances (SED) have not been adequately determined. Although various factors such as family functioning, heredity, diet, brain trauma or disorder, and stress have been suggested as possible causes (National Information Center for Children and Youth with Disabilities, 1997), research has not shown any of these factors to be a direct cause. Given the social and emotional nature of the defining characteristics of this disability, the ramifications in the areas of speech, language, and communication are evident, especially with communication. Social interactions, as defined by the appropriate use of pragmatics and vocabulary, are the greatest areas of need evidenced by students with serious emotional disturbances. Because language and communication are essential components of interpersonal relationships, children with SED may experience difficulties giving and receiving information from others. Consequently, language skills seem to affect children's social skills (Cullinan, Epstein, & Sabornie, 1992; Laughton & Hasenstab, 1986; McTear & Conti-Ramsden, 1992). Other ramifications in the speech and language sphere may be late onset of speech, idiosyncratic speech patterns, stream of irrelevant speech, lack of speech, abnormalities of loudness, pitch, or rhythm, self-talk, and aggressive or profane speech (Thomas & Carmack, 1990).

Activity

Observe in a school or your younger siblings, and listen to their interactions. Notice for clear speech pronunciations, voice clarity, fluency, and vocabulary development.

BOX 6.4 • *Considerations for Students with Serious Emotional Disabilities***

- Build upon existing communication systems and skills of students through observations of current communication strategies. Observe across settings, routines, and activities.
- Create a classroom climate of trust and respect, with opportunities for language stimulation and development.
- Teach vocabulary and words denoting emotional expression.
- Facilitate language development in naturalistic context settings, with intrinsically reinforcing activities. Build upon the desire to communicate with and interact with specific people and life activities that are motivating (lunchroom, interacting with peers, etc.)
- Facilitate the maximum use and reinforcement of the new language and communication skills. Collaborate with other team members, educators, family members, and peers that will assist this process.
- Use clearly presented rules and roles for all instruction, academic, behavioral, and language development. Set clear, observable expectations, teach and model, reinforce, and expect mastery of each of the goals as stated.
- Incorporate language into all aspects of the instruction. Reinforce and provide feedback and clarification immediately and consistently.
- Determine reinforcement and monitoring of the new communication and language skills.
- Ensure the maintenance and generalization of the new behavior through consistent monitoring across various settings.

**Activities synthesized from Gallagher, 1991; Mercer & Mercer, 1999; Oyer, Hall, & Haas, 1994; Sanger, Maag, & Shapera, 1994; Thomas & Carmack, 1990.

The educational implications and resulting programs for students with serious emotional disturbances need to include attention to mastering academics, developing social skills, and increasing self-awareness, self-control, and self-esteem. Within the academic domain, language impairments adversely impact a student's auditory comprehension, written expression, reading comprehension, mathematics, spelling, response to questions, basic concept development, and participation in class discussions (Camarata, Hughes, & Ruhl, 1988; Kamhi & Catts, 1989). Programs for instruction and remediation and specific instructional strategies in these academic areas will be similar to those created for students with learning disabilities, as the academic goals are similar (Fessler, Rosenberg, & Rosenberg, 1991).

In addition, it is very important to remember the basic premise of language and communication: interaction within a social setting. Aspects of pragmatics include understanding context, changing language and vocabulary for different purposes, and the use of appropriate social conventions for different settings (e.g., school, work, home, etc.). The use of verbal and nonverbal signals, turn-taking, initiating and maintaining conversations, and providing sufficient information are all aspects of conversational management and social competence (Brinton & Fujiki, 1989; Gallagher, 1991; Kirchner & Prutting, 1989; Laughton & Hasenstab, 1986). Given that, the resulting communication and language patterns and behaviors reveal much about the individual's perception of the environment and his or her relation with it. Assessment, instruction, and remediation should be based on clear goals and expectations established on the current needs of the individual student with SED within this social context (Maag, 1989), including the student's motivation, and self-image. This is especially critical when considering program goals to be achieved within the general education setting. The social setting, classroom rules, and behavioral and procedural expectations of the current setting and the inclusive setting must be clearly delineated, taught, and reinforced (Fuchs, Fernstrom, Scott, Fuchs, & Vandermeer, 1994). Social skills, communication and interpersonal skills, life space intervention (Long, 1991), problem-solving, and conflict-resolution techniques modeled, taught, and reinforced in a structured, consistent environment are an excellent language and communication curriculum.

> Appropriate communication with peers is also an important goal toward which to work; carefully structured situations for verbal interactions may improve interpersonal communication as well as speech and language skills. (Thomas & Carmack, 1990, p. 29)

The connection among academics, language, and social skills supports the need for the expanded involvement of the speech language pathologist with students with SED. "The speech pathologist can be a valuable member of the team that works with the student to expunge disorder and bring behavior into the normal range" (Thomas & Carmack, 1990, p. 29). The collaborative efforts of the speech-language pathologist and other special educators will continue to be beneficial for better addressing the needs of students (Bradshaw, Harn, & Ogletree, 1999).

Roles and Responsibilities of the Teacher

Given the philosophical framework of "how" children acquire language as the stage and the characteristics and educational implications of the "who" the students with disabilities are as the actors of this production, the stage manager orchestrates and facilitates the final production. Stage managers hold the vision of the successful final production. Their decisions and input are necessary for every aspect and every detail to ensure that the ultimate goals are achieved. They work in collaboration with numerous others, of various talents and skills, needing various levels of guidance and support.

Teachers, working collaboratively within a team, develop the vision and actualize its accomplishment for their students. It is the teacher who is the ultimate decision-maker and stage manager for the program development, curriculum decision, and instructional techniques and strategies used for each of the students. There is little doubt that teachers play a significant role in the lives of their students (Barth, 1990; Fenstermacher, 1989; McFarland, Fujiki, & Brinton, 1984). Garbee (1985, p. 75) was even more explicit, "The teacher greatly influences the development of a child who has a speech or language disorder."

When specifically considering a student with a speech or language disability, Oyer and colleagues (1994) discussed specific responsibilities of a teacher. The responsibilities are focused on three major concepts:

Awareness: The teacher needs to be knowledgeable about the student's specific and individual needs, both those within that classroom and those addressed within the IEP. The teacher also needs to be aware of the necessary services that are available to all students with disabilities, as well as the specific services that each individual student is currently receiving.

BOX 6.5 • *General Responsibilities of the Teacher*

- Be a Good Speech Model
- Create a Classroom Atmosphere Conducive for Communication
- Accept a Child with Communicative Problems
- Encourage Classmates to Accept a Child with Communicative Problems
- Consult and Collaborate with the Speech-Language Pathologist
- Detect Possible Communicative Problems and Make Appropriate Referrals to a Speech-language Pathologist
- Contribute to the Motivation of a Child
- Reinforce the Goals of Speech Therapy
- Help the Child Remember Therapy Appointments
- Help the Child Catch Up On What Is Missed in Speech therapy.

From Oyer, Hall, & Haas, 1994. Reprinted with permission.

Acceptance: The teacher must create, within the classroom, a climate of acceptance of students with disabilities. The classroom environment must be accepting of students at their current level of performance and conducive to communication and language development.

Advocacy: Whether to remind one of appointments or to plan instructional lessons that maximize each individual's language acquisition, the teacher constantly advocates for continued learning for each of the students. Teachers may also need to encourage for other students in the classroom to be more accepting of students with differing abilities. Through the efforts of the teacher, in collaboration with the speech-language pathologist, parents, administrators, and other educators, as necessary, students with disabilities do acquire and enhance their language.

Activity

Describe a model for instructional decision-making.

A Call to Action: Instructional Decision-Making

Because teachers are paramount in the classroom, the skills of the teacher as a decision-maker are critical to the instruction of language for students with disabilities. Teachers must be knowledgeable about research-based instructional practices and competently implement these practices and strategies, while consistently monitoring for student mastery of outcomes. Teachers need to be connoisseurs (Eisner, 1991) with a multitude of talents and depth of knowledge. To expertly address the needs of all students, but especially those with diverse learning needs, including those children with disabilities, a teacher must have a rich and varied knowledge base of foundational theories, instructional strategies, methods, and materials.

In addition, not only will teachers need to possess the knowledge and skills needed to teach language, but also teachers will need to thoughtfully apply this knowledge responsibly within the classroom. Based on the writings of Dewey (1933), and Schon (1983, 1987), the "teacher-as-technician" (Apple & Teitelbaum, 1985) is being replaced by a responsive and reflective "teacher-as-decision-maker." Shulman (1987, 1988) described teaching as a "continuing dialectic" within the classroom ecology. Therefore, to appropriately respond to the needs of the students within a classroom, teachers need *both* the deep knowledge base (connoisseurship) as well as the more complex skills of analysis and decision-making. Ysseldyke and colleagues (1992) saw this component as necessary to transform the image of "boss" who authoritatively ruled to "lead" teacher who facilitated learning. This revised role included "teacher-as-learner," in which there was questioning, as well as facilitating. Cochran-Smith and Lytle (1990) expanded the role of teacher as inquirer and "action researcher" to continue to be actively involved in the entire decision-making processes within classrooms while addressing the language needs of all students by thoughtfully and skill-fully implementing the necessary methods, materials, and strategies.

Activity

Observe a kindergarten classroom, a classroom for students with disabilities, and a high school English classroom. Identify the methods, materials and strategies implemented in all of the classrooms to develop language.

One model of an instructional decision process was developed by Dr. Floyd Hudson (1992) of the University of Kansas. It is an eight-step interactive and re-cursive process for instructional decision-making for classroom and individual student use. When planning for instruction for language acquisition, the process and the considerations remain basically similar. Whether planning a reading les-son in phonological awareness for the entire class of thirty students, a vocabulary lesson for seven students who are not reading at grade level, or for an individual student who receives instruction in a resource setting, the same planning process will occur.

- **Outcomes and Curriculum Goals and Objectives:** Covey (1989) suggested to "begin with the end in mind." Curriculum planning for instruction must begin with clearly delineated outcomes and goals for learning. Whether de-scribed by theorists and researchers, State Departments of Education, school districts, or members of an IEP team, the outcomes for students to be met through the language program must be clearly defined at the outset. If stu-dents with disabilities are to be included within the general classroom, grade-level expectations must be discussed as well as the outcomes for the students. Ultimately, what language skills (reading, writing, listening, speaking, social skills–pragmatics, etc.) will each of the students possess at the end of the in-structional period (year, week, day)? This knowledge provides the curricular framework for the instructional decision-making process.
- **Preskills:** Once knowledge of and agreement on the curricular framework have been identified, it is critical to determine the needs of the students within the context of the expectations. Whether assessed formally or infor-mally, as a class or as an individual, the next step in this decision-making pro-cess is the determination of the students' current knowledge of the particular skill. For example, if the curriculum outcome was silent reading comprehen-sion of a passage at the grade 5 level, knowledge of the student's current level of reading comprehension would be very important for appropriate plan-ning. In addition, this step in the instructional decision-making process also provides the opportunity to correct any incorrect prior knowledge of the topic to be taught. Once the preskills are assessed, there may be changes with

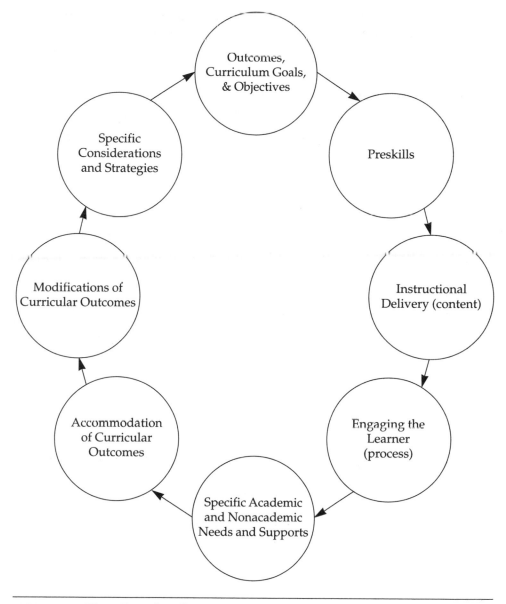

FIGURE 6.1   *Flow Chart for Effective Planning*
Little, 2000

the current planning for the class or for individual students as to the appropriateness of the stated outcomes for the individual students.

- **Instructional Delivery (Content):** The next two decisions really occur almost simultaneously: decisions about the content (what) and process (how) of instruction. Continuing the theater production metaphor, these two steps of the instructional decision-making are the script and staging notes for the actors as orchestrated by the stage manager. The teacher decides on the content of the continuously planned and implemented lessons that address the outcomes of the language curriculum. The specific teacher and learner objectives will be scripted for the time available. The necessary materials (props) must be readily available. What will the teacher *do* to facilitate the learning of the stated language content?

- **Engaging the Learner Research (Process):** Goodlad (1984) clearly shows the need to engage the learner within the lesson. Increasing academic learning time (Gage & Berliner, 1989) has direct positive benefits for student mastery of the stated outcomes. Therefore, at this point in the instructional process, decisions to engage the learner must be made. There are various models of instruction to consider (Joyce & Weil, 1983). For example, **direct instruction methods** (Bereiter & Englemann, 1966; Carnine, 1990; Gersten & Keating 1987) are advocated for skill development of relevant facts and concepts for students with disabilities and other students as well. With a specific six critical feature format, teachers demonstrate a skill, provide feedback to students as they practice the skill, and provide numerous examples and opportunities for students to practice the skills and generalize the skill to other settings.

  Another model of instruction is **cooperative learning.** Because of its success with heterogeneous groups and the interactive, yet independent, nature of this model, cooperative learning represents a viable approach to instructing students with diverse needs within a classroom structure (Johnson & Johnson, 1993; Slavin, 1986; 1990). Cooperative learning is an instructional arrangement in which small groups or teams of students work together to achieve a team and individual success in a way that promotes student responsibility (Mercer & Mercer, 1999).

  A third model of instruction is **class-wide peer tutoring** that combines the direct instruction and immediate feedback to students while in a cooperative, tutoring situation. Provided with materials and knowledge of the tutoring process, students within a classroom receive intensive, corrective feedback to the learner outcomes for the lesson. Research has proven excellent results in academic skills (e.g., spelling skills, reading decoding, and letter identification, etc.), while fostering improved self-esteem, developing appropriate social skills, and promoting positive interpersonal skills (Delquadri, Greenwood, Whorton, Carta, & Hall, 1986; Greenwood et al., 1988; Maheady, Sacca, & Harper, 1988). Not only are there other models of instruction that engage the students, but there are numerous active engagement techniques to use when instructing (e.g., manipulatives, wipe-off boards, choral responding, cueing, etc.). When deciding on the specific process to use, it is critical to ask:

  - *What will the students do to learn and to demonstrate mastery of the objectives for this lesson?*
  - *Will all of the students need this level of support? If not, then what other supports are needed by some of the students?*

- **Specific Academic and Nonacademic Needs and Supports:** There may be other goals associated with the lesson that may be an indirect, but very important, goal for lesson mastery. Some may be related to the lesson outcome, and some may not, for example, if the goal of a writing lesson is to write three complete sentences about a given topic. For most of the students, this task can be completed well. The lesson includes a graphic organizer to engage the students and provide a cognitive strategy and visual aid to organize the sentences. But what if three of the students in this second-grade class were born in Mexico and speak very little English? Planning must include contingencies for these students to complete the lesson goal, but with the necessary supports. Options might include a note-taker, if their oral language skills are developed. Picture words and Dolch words (most commonly used basic sights words in reading vocabulary) may be necessary to accommodate the needs of the learners as related to their current skill levels and the goals of the lesson. In addition, maybe two of the students are most successful in this class of thirty-two students if they receive written and verbal reinforcement according to the individual behavioral contracts. Three other students may need more immediate feedback, as this lesson is the first time they have completed sentences around a theme. Therefore, although planning has occurred with the framework of the curriculum and the preskills for the entire class, the knowledge of individual needs of students developing language skills is another critical component. Teachers will complete individual writing portfolios, specific skills rubrics, and/or checklists of mastered goals to organize these individual needs. Students can assist with this process, beginning in upper elementary school.

- **Accommodation of Curricular Outcomes:** In a general sense, accommodations are any adjustment or adaptation in the environment, instruction, or materials used for learning that enhances the student's participation within the learning activity (Udvari-Solner, 1993). In addition, an accommodation allows the individual to use his or her current skill repertoire while promoting the acquisition of new skills. The accommodations "level the playing field," providing the needed assistance for the student to achieve the goals of the lesson. A lesson written on an overhead or at the board would be much more challenging without glasses for those who need them to perform. Computer technology of word processors accommodates those students with a learning disability (spelling) who now can compose excellent sentences and compositions and need to only recognize the correct spelling. Accommodations can be described as seven types: **size, time, input, output, difficulty, participation,** and **level of support** (Ebeling, Deschenes, & Sprague, 1994). Any particular lesson can be adapted for any student with very specific needs within the classroom. For example, the writing lesson could be revised to accommodate students who, because of a disability, need more time to complete the three sentence paragraph. The list of accommodations is as varied as the needs of the student, the demands of the lesson goals, and the creativity of the teacher.

- **Modifications of the Curricular Outcomes:** Given the unique needs of some of the students with mild disabilities, it may be necessary to modify or change the goal of a lesson, either partially or completely. It is very important to differentiate between accommodations and modifications. At this stage of the planning process, the integrity of the agreed-on goals is being changed, adapted, or discarded completely. That fact must be clearly communicated to the team members who have been involved within the planning process. Students may be included in a classroom, but for very different goals. Goals of the lesson may be revised, but the same materials are used. For example, perhaps the lesson goal is to read and identify various parts of speech from a handout. An alternative goal might be for a student to highlight all of the initial sounds as identified on the same handout. Given the specific IEP goal for that student, that could be a realistic goal for the student with disabilities, and the student could learn and master this goal in a general education classroom, but this modification of lesson outcome and learner activity must be shared among all team members. At times, students could be learning a related language goal, but with completely different materials.
- **Evaluation by Outcomes:** The teaching process is not complete until the assessment of student learning has occurred. **Curriculum-based assessment** (Deno, 1987) refers to any approach that uses direct observation and recording of a student's performance in the school curriculum as a basis for obtaining information to make further instructional decisions. Evaluation of goals set for the entire grade level or any individual student may occur as appropriate. These data enable teachers to continue the instructional process of targeting new outcomes and goals for instruction. In addition, knowledge of results by the students has proven to reinforce continued learning by the students (Fuchs, Fuchs, & Hamlett, 1989).

Language Instruction: Specific Considerations and Strategies

Because language acquisition is an interactive process, the teacher should create an environment of communication within the classroom. Careful consideration to encourage language development throughout the day and within the classroom will be maximized through thoughtful planning. Considerations include:

- Literature books and high interest reading materials are displayed and available for student use;
- An abundance of writing materials, from crayons and paints to advanced computer word processing, is accessible;
- Interactive social settings to encourage appropriate verbal and nonverbal communication are built into the students' days;

- Instructional techniques that encourage discussions, role plays, cooperative groups, peer tutoring, debates, and so on are planned into every lesson; and
- Most importantly, the teacher believes that communication, language, and speech are acquired and mastered through continued practice and feedback across settings and is committed to actualize that belief.

Reflection

Why are teachers important within the instructional process?

As stated, language skills are developed in any interactive social setting. Therefore, any instructional classroom setting teaches language skills whether explicitly or implicitly. Lesson outcomes of report writing, planning and participating in a debate, speeches, writing answers to reading comprehension questions from a textbook, and so forth are but several examples of language outcomes. With integrated thematic instruction (Kovalik, 1994), units and lessons are planned around common themes across subject areas. Within these themes, specific outcomes and competencies are common, and, therefore, developed across each of the classes and/or subject areas. For example, the themes of problem-solving and conflict management can be developed and explored in the following areas:

History: Famous historical characters are often notorious due to their critical decisions. Complete a graphic organizer (compare/contrast chart or force-field analysis) of the issues for and against the critical decision. Discuss options and issues.

Science: The scientific method is a problem-solving approach to discovery. Apply to any experiments during this theme. Discuss logical steps when the hypothesis and/or process is not successful.

Math: Word problems are utilized for problem-solving. Try authentic examples (consumer math problems) and discuss next steps when the answer is not correct.

English: Debate a current issue from the evening news. Discuss both points of view or have students argue from the point of view opposed to their own. Discuss the pragmatics of debating, problem-solving, and conflict management. Possibly a specific problem-solving strategy could be shared throughout the team, grade level, or school.

Electives: Practice and reinforce the verbal and social skills of problem-solving and conflict management. Reinforce the use of the skills introduced and modeled in other classes.

In addition to areas of potential collaboration regarding content for language acquisition, when children with specific language disabilities are included within a classroom and the lesson outcomes are not primarily language acquisition (e.g., a ninth-grade U.S. history class), receptive and expressive language skills are needed by the students to be actively engaged with the learning. Mercer and Mercer (1999) reviewed the current research to provide strategies that are helpful to teachers who facilitate the learning for students with disabilities in language.

> *Reflection*
>
> **What are several characteristics of students with mild disabilities (mental retardation, learning disabilities, and serious emotional disturbances)?**

Specific Lessons and Ideas

This last section of the chapter will focus on a brief review of the instructional implications of the discreet components of language: (Form) phonology, morphology, syntax and (Content) semantics and pragmatics. Each of these language components may present areas for instruction or remediation as outcomes and goals for the class or any individual student. This will depend on the curricular expectations and the language development of the particular student(s). Several lessons in each area will be considered that can be adapted or modified based on the instructional outcomes for the lesson and the developmental needs of the students (see previous section on instructional decision-making).

Phonology

Phonology is the study of the rules governing speech-sound production. In contrast, **phonetics** is the study of the way speech sounds are articulated, and **phonics** is the system by which symbols represent sounds in the alphabetic system (Adams, Foorman, Lundberg, & Beeler, 1998). There has been much discussion in the literature about the methods and approaches used for initial reading instruction, which includes these areas in language acquisition of sound production. (See Chapter 4 for further discussion.)

Specific goals in phonology and articulation should be developed in collaboration with the speech-language pathologist and involve the parents because phonological rules contain speech-sound production that have biological and environmental reasons. Biological concerns are due to the limitations of the articulatory system of the student. Regional and environmental feedback to sound production also will impact the precise articulation of the phonemes.

Phonemes are the units of speech that are represented by the letters of an alphabetic system. "Conscious awareness of phonemes is distinct from the built-in sensitivity that supports speech production and reception. It is this sort of explicit, reflective knowledge that falls under the rubric of *phonemic awareness*" (Adams,

BOX 6.6 • *Strategies to Assist Language Comprehension (Receptive Language)*

1. If student frequently has difficulty following directions or understanding information of increased complexity, establish eye contact and maintain attention before presenting information. Cue the student to listen through the use of silent pauses or instructions or look at the teacher (Mercer & Mercer, 1999).

2. Use introductory statements (e.g., "These are the five main points," "Before we begin, you need your homework on your desk.") to provide an organizational framework and help students prepare for a task (Mercer and Mercer, 1999).

3. Present new concepts using as many modalities as possible (e.g., auditory, visual, and kinesthetic), and use gestures to augment verbal presentations (Bos & Vaughn, 1988).

4. To increase understanding of the relationship between semantic role and word order, encourage students to act out, draw, discuss, etc. the task (Connell, 1986).

5. Explain and demonstrate active listening skills (e.g., think, look at the speaker, repeat to yourself, etc.) (Chabon & Prelock, 1989).

6. To enhance student's recall and memory of vocabulary, use various mnemonics and memory devices in which the new words are associated with a new word or concept (Mastropieiri, Scruggs, & Fulk, 1990).

7. Instruct using semantic or graphic organizers that cluster key information of related main ideas and provide a verbal (semantic) and graphic organizer for acquisition of information (Pehrsson & Denner, 1988).

Strategies to Assist Language Production (Expressive Language)

1. Teach language in various natural settings and in connection with other curriculum content (Wig & Semel, 1984)

2. Model good language skills, and ask students to imitate what they hear (Connell, 1986).

3. Use structured language programs that provide adequate opportunities to practice a new skill as well as interactive opportunities to practice the skill in relevant contexts (Bos & Vaughn, 1988).

4. When students have difficulty with word retrieval, examine the setting and indices such as response time, error patterns, and substitutions.

5. Use semantic maps and organizers to improve a student's retrieval skills for sounds, words, and concepts, such as categorizing or classifying words.

6. Teach generalization of language skills through three phases: (1) an orientation phase in which the student becomes aware of the different contexts applicable, (2) an activation phase in which the practice is provided in a variety of situations, and (3) a maintenance phase in which periodic probes are conducted to ensure proficiency is maintained.

Adapted from: Mercer, C., & Mercer, A. (1999). *Teaching Students with Learning Problems.* Englewood Cliffs, NJ: Merrill.

Foorman, Lundberg, & Beeler, 1998, p. 3). There is much currently written and researched in this area of phonemic awareness and a multitude of materials are available (Adams, Foorman, Lundberg, & Beeler, 1998; Fitzpatrick, 1997; Scott, 1998; Torgesen, 1996).

Sample Lessons: Outcomes and Abbreviated Summary

- **Syllable Counting:** Have students repeat names of familiar objects while clapping, tapping, or rapping out the number of syllables in unison.
- **Phoneme Isolation:** Each child receives a smile face to attach to his or her thumb. Each time the student hears a specific phoneme identified, the child then gives the "thumbs up" to the sound. Variation: Ask for specific sounds in various locations: initial, medial, ending.
- **Phoneme Blending:** With several items in a "mystery box," have students guess the items using phoneme clues.
- **Phoneme Counting:** With a bag of items, chart paper, and a marker, the students identify and categorize each of the mystery items as to the correct number of phonemes and place the item on the correct place on the chart paper (e.g., a picture of a key would be placed under the number 2 for the correct number of phonemes).
- **Phoneme Substitution and Blending:** With alphabet cards and a pocket chart, create new one-syllable words by substituting various phonemes.

Morphology

Morphology deals with the prefixes and suffixes that are added to words in order to change meaning (Oyer, Hall, & Haas, 1994). A morpheme is the smallest unit of meaning in a language. A free morpheme may be used alone, as it has meaning (e.g., *friend, my, all,* etc.). However, a bound morpheme has a specific meaning but must be attached to a free morpheme to have meaning. For example, in the English language, one of the functions of the morpheme *-s* is to indicate plural. Other examples of commonly used morphemes include: *-er, -est, -less, -un,* and *-ship.* Areas of morphology that may need instruction and remediation are in the areas of comparison and contrast, plurals, irregular word forms, and time and tense indicators.

Sample Lessons: Outcomes and Abbreviated Summary

- **Comparatives:** Using manipulative or picture cards, have students arrange in order from "smallest" to "tallest," "oldest" to "youngest," and any other comparative indicators.
- **Number:** Divide the students into two groups. Alternating teams, one member says, "I see a _____" (noun). A member from the second team must see two of the object, correctly repeating the sentence with the correct plural form of the word.
- **Case and Gender:** Prepare cards with pronouns that are subjective, objective, and possessive. With sentences written on the board, have students replace the nouns with the appropriate pronoun, matching case and gender.

- **Tense:** On a large piece of chart paper, write "YESTERDAY," TODAY," and "TOMORROW." Say a sentence, and select a student; ask him or her to stand in front of a piece of chart paper and repeat the sentence for that specific tense. ("Yesterday, I went to the store." "Today I am going to the store." "Tomorrow, I will go to the store.")

Syntax

The syntactic component of a language consists of the rules for ordering words in such a way that the speaker can be understood. Grammatical rules state the appropriate word orderings for our intended meanings. Rules also signal the transformation of one sentence construction into another so that compound sentences, negatives, questions, passives, imperatives, and sentences with embedded clauses can be produced (Oyer, Hall, & Haas, 1994). Developmentally, students may not understand the passive voice, a transformation, until their early teens (Horgan, 1978). The more complicated the sentence constructions, the more a student with language disabilities with syntax may lose the meaning of the sentence. Additionally, the student may not be able to express his or her needs within the sentence constructions that he or she can use. Using concrete and authentic examples may be the best way to begin instruction or remediation. The University of Kansas Center for Research on Learning developed strategies that explicitly teach language skills in this area, especially for adolescents.

Sample Lessons: Outcomes and Abbreviated Summary
- **Sentence Transformation through Paraphrasing.** With specific materials developed at the University of Kansas, students are taught the "RAP Strategy:"
  - R—Read a passage
  - A—Ask yourself questions about the meaning
  - P—Put the meaning in your own words
- **Sentence Combining/Complex Sentence Formation.** With individual word cards of specific conjunctions and sentence strips of simple sentences, encourage the students to create their own complex sentences. Encourage the correct written expressions of the new complex sentences by writing the new sentences on the board/paper.
- **Questions about Questions.** Place the name of an item in a secret place. Have students ask "20 Questions" to determine the actual item chosen. Variation: The students can restate the question as a simple sentence, an imperative, an exclamation, and so on.
- **Sequencing and Ordering Information Correctly.** With materials needed to make a peanut butter and jelly sandwich, have students write the exact directions on paper. One at a time, ask another student to demonstrate the directions as written and sequenced.

Semantics

Semantics is the meaning and multiple meanings of words (vocabulary) and word combinations produced by the syntactic rules. Words provide the code to label and refer to the environment. We cannot adequately interact without the ability to call and recall the specific labels of common meaning that the words provide. The first words we learn are concrete, but our language becomes more abstract as we acquire skill. During their school years, and in particular, adolescence, children also increase their ability to use and to understand figurative language (Nippold, 1993; Owens, 1984), words used as puns, idioms, similes, metaphors, proverbs, and sarcasm. Figurative language requires a great command of the language, not only the literal sense, but also the social connotations that add to the meanings of some forms of figurative language. Students with some types of language disabilities, like aphasia, may have difficulty recalling the exact word. In other cases, the multiple meanings of words will be a source of difficulty as well. Much exposure to various vocabulary, both literal and figurative, is very important to instruction and remediation within the area of semantics.

Sample Lessons: Outcomes and Abbreviated Summary
- **Multiple Meaning.** Given sentence strips of multiple meanings, the student selects one and acts out at least two different meanings for the sentence as written, for example, "The sailor kept the watch," "Dad smoked a turkey for dinner," and "Describe the victim's state." Encourage the students to create their own and/or illustrate their multiple answers.
- **Figurative Language.** Have students describe and draw various similes such as "Quiet as a mouse," "Slow as a turtle," "Hungry as a horse." Have them complete a T-Chart, including, "What does this look like?" "What does this sound like?"
- **Cause and Effect.** With prepared cause-and-effect sentence strips, have students match the cause with the effect. For example, "I studied a lot" with "I made an 'A' on the test."
- **Prepositional Phrases.** Create an obstacle course. Have students complete the course, while responding to prepositions, such as *over, under, to, around, underneath, with, without,* and so on.

Pragmatics

Pragmatics refers to the rules for language use in a social context for a particular purpose. The emphasis on pragmatics has been relatively recent in comparison to the other components of language (Oyer, Hall, & Haas, 1994). Given the importance of being able to interact within one's social setting, however, it has been called the area of the most important language growth both during the school-age and adult years. Adults most often lose their employment because they lack social skills, certainly the emphasis on the pragmatics of language is very important.

Reflection

Name and describe the five components of language and the characteristics of each.

Another important pragmatic aspect of language is the ability of students to use language to gain entry into and maintain their position within a peer group. They do so by using the current and correct slang expressions and employing other appropriate verbal and nonverbal strategies with their peers (Nippold, 1993). Pragmatics embodies the entire communication process, as stated and unstated; verbal and nonverbal communication norms must be adhered to in each given social setting.

- What is the precise language to be used?
- How quickly do people speak?
- What are all of the nuances of various interpersonal, nonverbal gestures?
- What is the correct body posture?
- When should one respond to questions?

Students with disabilities, especially in the area of social skills, may not know, use, and distinguish the appropriate social skills for the context. Explicit use of social skills and pragmatics and encouraging them to generalize the skills across numerous social settings is critical to students with disabilities.

Sample Lessons: Outcomes and Abbreviated Summary
- **Prosodic Features of Mood and Meaning.** Select an interesting but simple play for the students to act out in various ways. Discuss the meanings of the play and the feelings of the actors.
- **Kinesics.** Find pictures that display various emotions and discuss the meanings of the facial features and emotions with the students. Have the students imitate and role-play. (Use of a video camera could be helpful here.)
- **Proxemics.** Have students practice a "six-inch voice" for their cooperative learning groups for class. They can measure the space and practice the loudness of their voice that would then be appropriate. Encourage further discussions regarding the same idea in different settings, e.g., hallways, playground, hospital, and so on.

Reflection

What are some considerations for instructional programming for all students with disabilities in the area of language acquisition and development?

Summary

This chapter discussed some of the considerations in developing and implementing language programs for students with disabilities. Specific information about students with disabilities that may impact language development was also discussed. It is important to note that speech, language, and communication skills are developed through direct and indirect interactions in all of our social settings. Further, each child is unique in his or her language abilities. Any intervention should be individualized and designed to meet the needs of the individual student. Categorical description of these students is not intended to result in self-fulfilling prophecies, but rather as an informational guide that will assist you in meeting some of the needs of the students in your classroom. It is our hope that, with this information, you will also have a better knowledge of the language characteristics and interventions so that you will be better prepared to serve them in inclusive settings.

References and Suggested Readings

Adams, M. J., Foorman, B., Lundberg, I., & Beeler, T. (1998). *Phonemic awareness in young children.* Baltimore, MD: Brookes.

Apple, M., & Teitelbaum, K. (1985). Are teachers losing control of their jobs? *Social Education, 49*(5), 372–375.

Balius, F. A., & Bauer, M. S. (1995). Storytelling: Integrating therapy and curriculum for students with serious emotional disturbances. *TEACHING Exceptional Children, 27,* 24–28.

Barth, R. (1990). *Improving schools from within.* San Francisco, CA: Jossey Bass, Inc.

Bereiter, C., & Englemann, S. E. (1966). *Teaching disadvantaged children in the preschool.* Englewood Cliffs, NJ: Prentice-Hall.

Bos, C. S., & Vaughn, S. (1988). *Strategies for teaching students with learning and behavior problems.* Boston: Allyn & Bacon.

Bradshaw, M. L., Harn, W. E., & Ogletree, B. T. (1999). The speech-language pathologist in the schools: Changing roles. *Intervention in School and Clinic, 34*(3), 163–169.

Braine, M. (1971). *On two types of the internalization of grammar.* New York: Academic Press.

Brinton, B., & Fujiki, M. (1989). *Conversational management with language impaired children: Pragmatic assessment and intervention.* Rockville, MD: Aspen.

Brinton, B., & Fujiki, M. (1998). Participation in cooperative learning activities by *Research,* children with specific language impairment.

Journal of Speech, Language, & Hearing 41, 1193–1206.

Camarata, S., Hughes, C., & Ruhl, K. (1988). Mild/moderate behaviorally disordered students: A population at-risk for language disorders. *Language, Speech, and Hearing Services in Schools, 19,* 199–200.

Carnine, D. (1990). Beyond technique—Direct instruction and higher order skills. *Direct Instruction News, 9*(3), 1–13.

Chabon, S. S., & Prelock, P. A. (1989). Strategies of a different stripe: Our response to a zebra question about language and its relevance to the school curriculum. *Seminars in Speech and Language, 10,* 241–251.

Chomsky, N. A. (1965). *Aspects of the theory of syntax.* Cambridge, MA: MIT Press.

Chomsky, N. A. (1994). *Language development.* Cambridge, MA: MIT Press.

Cochran-Smith, M., & Lytle, S. (1990). Research on teaching and teacher research: The issues that divide. *Educational Researcher, 3,* 2–10.

Cole, K. N., Coggins, T. E., & Vanderstoep, C. (1999). The influence of language/cognitive profile on discourse intervention outcome. *Language, Speech, and Hearing Services in Schools, 30,* 61–67.

Connell, P. J. (1986). Acquisition of semantic role by language-disordered children: Differences between production and comprehension. *Journal of Speech and Hearing Research, 29,* 366–374.

Covey, S. (1989). *The seven habits of highly effective people.* New York: Simon Schuster.

Cullinan, D., Epstein, M. H., Sabornie, E. J. (1992). Selected characteristics of a national sample of seriously emotionally disturbed adolescents. *Behavioral Disorders, 17,* 273–280.

Delquadri, J., Greenwood, C. R., Whorton, D., Carta, J. J., and Hall, R. V. (1986). Classwide peer tutoring. *Exceptional Children, 52*(6), 535–542.

Deno, S. L. (1987). Curriculum-based measurement. *Teaching Exceptional Children, 20*(1), 41–42.

Deshler, D., Ellis, E., & Lenz, B. (1996). Teaching adolescents with learning disabilities: *Strategies and methods* (2nd ed.) Denver: Love.

Deshler, D. D., & Schumaker, J. (1987). Learning strategies: An instructional alternative for low-achieving adolescents. *Exceptional Children, 52,* 583–590.

Dewey, J. (1933). *How we think.* New York: Heath.

Dixon, M. E., & Rossi, J. C. (1995). Directors of their own learning: A reading strategy for students with learning disabilities. *Teaching Exceptional Students, 27,* 11–14.

Drew, C. J., Hardman, M. L., & Logan, D. R. (1996). *Mental retardation. A life cycle approach* (6th ed.). Englewood Cliffs, NJ: Merrill/Prentice-Hall.

Ebeling, D. G., Deschenes, C., & Sprague, J. (1994). *Adapting curriculum and instruction in inclusive classrooms.* Bloomington, IN: Institute for the Study of Developmental Disabilities.

Eisener, E. (1991). *The enlightened eye: Qualitative inquiry and the enhancement of educational practice.* New York: Macmillan.

ERIC Clearinghouse on Disabilities and Gifted Education, *ERIC Digest.* Reston, VA: ED 38509595.

Fenstermacher, G. (1989). The place of science and epistemology in Schon's conceptional of reflective practice. In P. Grimmett & G. Erickson (Eds.), *Reflection in teacher education* (pp. 39–46). New York: Teachers College Press.

Fessler, M. A., Rosenberg, M. S., & Rosenberg, L. A. (1991). Concomitant learning disabilities and learning problems among students with behavior/emotional disorders. *Behavior Disorders, 16,* 97–106.

Fitzpatrick, J. (1997). *Phonemic awareness.* Cypress, CA: Creative Teaching Press.

Frost, J., & Emery, M. (1995). Academic interventions for dyslexic children with phonological core deficits.

Fuchs, D., Fernstrom, P., Scott, S., Fuchs, L., & Vandermeer, L. (1994). Classroom ecological inventory: A process for mainstreaming. *TEACHING Exceptional Children, 26*(3), 11–15.

Fuchs, D., & Fuchs, L. (1994). Inclusive schools movement and the radicalization of special education reform. *Exceptional children, 60*(4), 294–309.

Fuchs, L. S., Fuchs, D., and Hamlett, C. L. (1989). Effects of instructional use of curriculum-based measurement to enhance instruction programs. *Remedial and Special Education 10*(2), 43–52.

Gage, N. & Berliner, D. (1989). Nurturing the critical, practical, and artistic thinking of teachers. *Phi Delta Kappan, 70*(3), 212–214.

Gallagher, T. M. (1991). *Pragmatics of language: Clinical practice issues.* San Diego, CA: Singular.

Garbee, F. E. (1985). The speech-language pathologist as a member of the educational team. In R. J. Van Hattum (Ed.), *Organization of speech-language services in schools* (pp. 58–129). San Diego, CA: College-Hill Press.

Gersten, R., & Keating, T. (1987). Long-term benefits from direct instruction. *Educational Leadership, 44*(6), 28–31.

Goodlad, J. (1984). *A place called school: Prospects for the future.* New York: McGraw-Hill.

Greenwood, C. R., Carta, J. J., & Hall, R. V. (1988). The use of peer tutoring strategies in classroom management and educational instruction. *School Psychology Review, 17*(2), 258–275.

Highnam, C., Wegmann, J., & Woods, J. (1999). Visual and verbal metaphors among children with typical language disorders. *Journal of Communication Disorders, 32* (1), 25–35.

Horgan, D. (1978). The development of the full passive. *Journal of Child Language, 5,* 65–80.

Hudson, F. (1992). Personal Communication.

Individuals with Disabilities Education Act (PL 97-103). US Congress. Washington, DC: Author.

Johnson, D. W., & Johnson, R. (1989). *Cooperation and competition.* Edina, MN: Interaction Books.

Joyce, B., & Weil, S. (1983). *Models of instruction.* New York: McGraw Hill.

Kagan, S. (1990). The structural approach to cooperative learning. *Educational Leadership, 47*(4), 12–15.

Kamhi, A. G., & Catts, H. W. (Eds.). (1989). *Reading disabilities: A developmental language perspective.* Boston: College Hill Press.

Kirchner, D. M., & Prutting, C. A. (1989). Pragmatic criteria for communicative competence. *Seminars in speech and language, 10,* 42–50.

Kovalik, S. (1994). *ITI: The model.* Kent, WA: Books for Educators.

Laughton, J., & Hasenstab, M. S. (1986). *The language learning process: Implications for management of disorders.* Rockville, MD: Aspen.

Lenneberg, E. H. (1967). *Biological foundations of language.* New York: Wiley.

Long, N. J. (1991). *Teaching children with behavior disorders.* Columbus, OH, Merrill.

Maag, J. W. (1989). Assessment of social skills training: Methodological and conceptual issues for research and practice. *Remedial and Special Education, 10* (4), 6–17.

Maag, J. W., Sanger, D., & Shapera, N. R. (1994). Language problems among students with emotional and behavioral disorders. *Intervention in School and Clinic, 30* (2), 103–107.

Maheady, L., Sacca, M. K., & Harper, G. F. (1988). Classwide peer tutoring with mildly handicapped high school students. *TEACHING Exceptional Children, 55,* 52–59.

Mastropieri, M. A., Scruggs, T. E., & Fulk, B. J. M. (1990). Teaching abstract vocabulary with the keyword methods: Effects on recall and comprehension. *Journal of Learning Disabilities, 23,* 92–97, 107.

McDounough, K. M. (1989). Analysis of the expressive language characteristics of emotionally handicapped students in social interactions. *Behavioral Disorders, 14* (2), 127–139.

McFarland, S. C., Fujiki, M., & Brinton, B. (1984). *Coping with communication handicaps.* San Diego, CA: College Hill Press.

McLean, J. E., & Snyder-McLean, L. K. (1978). *A transactional approach to early language training.* New York: Merrill/Macmillan.

McTear, M. F., & Conti-Ramsden, G. (1992). *Pragmatics disability in children.* San Diego, CA: Singular.

Mercer, C., & Mercer, A. (1999). *Teaching students with learning problems.* Englewood Cliffs, NJ: Merrill. National Information Center for Children and Youth with Disabilities. Author. (1996).

National Information Center for Children and Youth with Disabilities (1997). General information about learning disabilities. Fact Sheet Number 7. Washington, DC: Author.

Nippold, M. A. (1993). Developmental markers in adolescents: Syntax, semantics, and pragmatics. *Language, Speech, and Hearing Services in the Schools, 24,* 21–29.

Ostrosky, M. M., Drasgow, E., & Halle, J. W. (1999). "How can I help you get what you want? A communication strategy for students with severe disabilities." *TEACHING Exceptional Children, 31,* 56–61.

Owens, R. E. (1984). *Language development: An introduction.* Columbus, OH: Charles E. Merrill.

Oxford, R. (1990). *Language learning strategies: What every teacher should know.* Boston: Heinle and Heinle.

Oyer, H. J., Hall, B. J., & Haas, W. H. (1994). *Speech, language, and hearing disorders: A guide for the teacher.* Boston: Allyn & Bacon.

Pehrsson, R. S., & Denner, P. R. (1988). Semantic organizers: Implications for reading and writing. *Topics in Language Disorders, 8* (3), 4–32.

Richards, J. C. (1990). *The language teaching matrix.* New York: Cambridge University Press.

Sanger, D., Maag, J. W., and Shapera, N. R. (1994). Language problems among students with emotional and behavioral disorders. *Intervention in School and Clinic, 30,* 103–108.

Schon, D. (1983). *The reflective practitioner: How practitioners think in action.* New York: Basic Books.

Schon, D. (1987). *Educating the reflective practitioner: Toward a new design for teaching and learning in the professions.* San Francisco, CA: Jossey-Bass.

Scott, V. G. (1998). *Phonemic awareness: Lessons, games, and activities to teach phonemic awareness.* McPherson, KS: Author.

Shaywitz, S. E. (1996, November). Dyslexia. *Scientific American,* 98–104.

Shulman, L. (1987). Knowledge and teaching: foundations of the new reform. *Harvard Educational Review, 57*(1), 1–21.

Shulman, L. (1988). The dangers of dichotomous thinking in education. In P. Grimmett & G. Erickson (Eds.), *Reflection in teacher education.* New York: Teachers College Press.

Slavin, R. (1986). *Using student team learning* (3rd ed.). Baltimore, MD: Center for Research on Elementary and Middle Schools, Johns Hopkins University.

Slavin, R. (1990). Research on cooperative learning: Consensus and controversy. *Educational Leadership, 47* (4), 52–54.

Staats, A. (1971). Linguistic—mentalistic theory versus an explanatory S—R learning theory of language development. In D. L. Slobin (Ed.), *The ontogenesis of grammar.* New York: Academic Press.

Thomas, P. J., & Carmack, F. F. (1990). *Speech and language: Detecting and correcting special needs.* Boston: Allyn & Bacon.

Torgesen, J. (1996). Phonological awareness. Florida State Board of Education: Author.

Udvari-Solner, A. (1993). *Curricular adaptations: Accommodating the instructional needs of diverse learners in the context of general education.* Kansas State Board of Education: Author.

Wig, E. H., & Semel, E. M. (1984). *Language assessment and intervention for the learning disabled* (2nd ed.). New York: Merrill/Macmillan.

Wolk, L., & Meisler, A. W. (1998). Phonological assessment: A systematic comparison of conversation and picture naming. *Journal of Communication Disorders, 31* (4), 291–313.

Ysseldyke, J., Algozzine, R., & Thurlow, M. (1992). *Critical issues in special education.* Boston: Houghton Mifflin.

7

Problems of Phonology/Articulation: Identification and Remediation

Martha S. Lue

Chapter Objectives _____

On completion of the chapter, the reader will be able to:

- Identify the most common types of phonological/articulation problems;
- Specify causal factors; and
- Identify assessment instruments, interventions, and strategies that the classroom teacher might use in the areas of phonology and articulation.

- Twelve middle-school students classified as language/learning disordered were working on their story board presentations. After writing a story and drawing action frame pictures, students were asked to present their stories orally in front of the class. (By definition, students with language/learning disorders must qualify for placement in a class for severe language and learning disabilities.) As the students presented their stories orally, the presenters were consistently given encouraging comments from their teacher and the assistant, "excellent eye contact, wonderful pictures, now put the poster down so that your peers can see your face; when you see the period at the end of the sentence, stop, take a pause, and look at your audience." This session of the class is being cotaught by the speech-language pathologist and the classroom teacher. The classroom teacher has an advanced degree in speech-language pathology and special education. Turn-taking, appropriate posture, and pragmatics were stressed in the presentations. Over 90 percent of the youngsters presented phonological processing difficulties, such as listening comprehension, oral expression, and difficulty in putting sounds together when reading. The coteaching arrangement is working very well and is considered a model for the local school district.

- The child was referred for an in-depth language evaluation as a part of the three-year reevaluation process for students in the exceptional education program. The child attends a local elementary school and receives services from both the programs for children who are specifically learning disabled as well as for those demonstrating deficits in speech/language. The purpose of this reevaluation was to assess any changes in language functioning in comprehension, verbal expressive skills, and survival communication skills.

  The child's mother completed a ***Speech-Language Questionnaire for Parents.*** The mother shared that the child's greatest problems were those of paying attention and following through with directions. Further, the mother said that the child did not talk very much to people in school and that the child was very shy. Other areas addressed in the evaluation included:

  Verbal/cognitive. The child had significant difficulty with the vocabulary tasks of understanding figurative language and words with multiple meanings.

  Language comprehension/listening skills. The child presented weak abilities in processing information and following directions as noted previously by her mother and teacher.

  Language production/conversational skills. Phonology: No significant problems presented; no intervention necessary.

  Syntax/morphology. On the ***Clinical Evaluation of Language Fundamentals (rev.),*** the child rated "severe" in sentence assembly and recalling sentences.

  Semantics. On the ***Expressive One-Word Picture Vocabulary Test,*** a raw score of 88 was achieved, with a standard score of 98, and a stanine of five.

Language sample analysis. The child has difficulties in vocabulary and understanding, but expressive word meanings were observed.

Pragmatics. The child exhibited moderate difficulties in planning what to say, sequencing in a logical manner, and in producing grammatically correct sentences. Mild difficulties in pitch, volume, and quality of voice were observed.

Results indicated that the child has made steady progress in her academic efforts, but still shows significant weaknesses that will affect her ability to have her needs adequately met. She continues to show a need for increased speech/language services and should be considered for placement in a language/learning disordered class.

- At first, the nine-year-old boy was reluctant to speak in the classroom. When called on by the teacher, he simply said quietly, "I don't know," or he shook his head. When he did speak, he often spoke in whispered tones, and could only be heard by those close to him. After further efforts at engaging the child in communicating, the classroom teacher accurately observed that the child's speech exhibited one of the most common communication problems found in school-age children, an articulation problem. Errors exhibited in his speech included substitutions and omissions of sounds. For example, he frequently substituted the sound /t/ for /k/ and /w/ for /r/. Instead of saying the word *cake,* he'd say the word *take.* Instead of saying the word *red,* he'd say the word *wed.* Omissions at the beginning and ending of words were also observed. He was referred to the speech-language pathologist for testing. Results of the evaluation indicated an articulation problem. The child began articulation group therapy twice a week, for thirty minutes. Conversely, the speech pathologist worked closely with the classroom teacher to ensure that the skills learned in the therapy setting were generalized to the classroom and to the home setting. The mother is very excited about the child's progress. He appears more confident in speaking and even agreed to join a scout troop that reads to Head Start children.

The vignettes presented describe the perplexity and complexity of the phonological/ articulation process. While a previous chapter dealt with the normal development of speech and language in depth, this chapter will focus primarily on various types of phonological/articulation problems, causal factors, assessment instruments, and interventions that teachers might use. The descriptions, although not exhaustive, should serve as an impetus to one's own "strategies" list.

It is important that classroom teachers understand this topic, for most students will exhibit some type of language or learning problem. Phonological disorders are among the most common types of communication problems found in school-age children. Difficulties may range from problems in phonology to pragmatics. Other difficulties might include word-retrieval problems, echolalia, and articulation problems identified with syndromes or those associated with differing cultural/linguistic backgrounds.

Language Parameters

Humans have an innate biological basis for hearing and producing sounds (Gleason, 1993). This basis is then shaped by language experiences, including cognitive reactions to articulatory challenges. Further, oral language is a learned behavioral system that enables people to transmit their ideas and culture from generation to generation (Mercer & Mercer, 1989). One cannot fully appreciate human speech unless one understands the sound system from which specific phonemes are drawn to make up spoken words (Hulit & Howard, 1993). It is this study of speech sounds, rules that determine how sounds can be sequenced into syllables and words, that we call *phonology*.

Spoken language is made up of parameters or components. It is generally accepted that spoken language is divided into five components or parameters. As described in previous chapters, these components/parameters include:

- phonology: sound system of the language; rules governing the structure of syllables and words;
- morphology: rules governing change in meaning;
- syntax: word order;
- semantics: word meaning, word content rules, grammatical rules;
- pragmatics: language use within a communication context.

Reed (1994) adds that these components are all part of a system, and "are therefore governed by regularities and sets of rules that all speakers of a specific language must learn, if they are to communicate effectively." Bloom and Lahey (1978) classify these components as:

- form (phonology, morphology, syntax)
- content (semantics)
- usage (pragmatic)

Language development does not occur in isolation, but combined with other aspects of child development. For the purpose of this chapter, emphasis will be placed on phonological development and disorders. Later material will cover cultural influences on language.

Phonology versus Articulation

Phonology and articulation are closely related, and the distinction between what the two terms refer to is often difficult to describe. Sometimes they are used interchangeably. *Phonology,* is both a form of language—is the sound system of a language and the linguistic rules that govern possible sound combinations in that language (ASHA, 1982)—and it is also the study of the rules for using the sounds of a language. *Articulation* "is the process by which sounds, syllables, and words are formed when the tongue, jaw, teeth, lips, and palate alter the airstream coming from the vocal folds, when forming sounds, syllables, and words" (ASHA, 1996). A more detailed discussion of these two terms will be handled later in the chapter.

The Phonological System

The phonological system interfaces with the semantic and syntactic components to result in language—a symbolic social system (Bernstein & Tiegerman, 1993). All children learning a language acquire the phonemes of a language in an ordered and predictable sequence (Shelton, 1995a). The following represents a traditional discussion of the phonological system. Topics to be covered include phonology, phonemes, and phonetics.

Phonology

One sense of the term *phonology* denotes the sound system of a language. The sound system in English comprises consonants, vowels, and diphthongs. Moreover, phonology concerns the relationship among the speech sounds of a language, including the phonetic resemblances due to the way that they are produced. Three aspects of phonological development have been identified: (1) the way a sound is stored in a child's mind; (2) the way a sound is actually said by the child; and (3) the rules and processes that relate the two (Bowen, 1999). Speech sounds are acquired in an orderly sequence through about the seventh year. Children, add Eisenson and Ogilvie (1983), begin their phonological development as early as nine months, discriminating among phonemes according to broad categories, that is, stops, fricatives, affricates, liquids, glides, and so forth.

Phonemes

A *phoneme* is the smallest unit of language. It is a linguistic unit significantly different from all other sounds within a language system. In the English language, there are approximately forty-five phonemes—vowels, consonants, and diphthongs. However, the number may vary, depending on a number of factors, including regional dialect, classification system, and speaker idiosyncrasies (Weiss & Lillywhite, 1981).

Phonetics

Phonetics, as defined by Vergason & Anderegg (1997) refers to "the study of speech sound words involving the breakdown of into separate said elements." It is the study of the speech sounds made by the human vocal apparatus and their acoustic output.

Activity

Review three current journals in the area of phonology (e.g., *Language, Speech, and Hearing Services in the Schools*). Summarize the articles and include your own thoughts using the 3-R approach—Reaction, Relevance, and Responsibility.

Young Children and Phonological Awareness

Researchers note that young children's phonological awareness abilities are excellent predictors of later reading and spelling performance levels. Further, children with poor phonological awareness experience greater difficulty learning to read (Hulit & Howard, 1993).

The child's first word is usually spoken at around one year of age. By one-and-a-half years, many children use about fifty words and are beginning to make two-word sentences. "Adultlike" speech is evident by age four, and "adult standard speech" appears by age seven. Factors that may identify possible phonological disorders include:

- Delays of six months or more;
- Consistency of deviation, stimulability, and overall intelligibility; and
- Whether the level of communicative ability is appropriate for a child's age.

Other indicators may include the number of speech sounds in error, consistency of misarticulations, frequency of occurrence of error sounds, phonological processes used, pitch inflection, voice quality, and fluency (Gordon-Brannon, 1994).

Phonological Processing

To fully comprehend the concept of phonological processing, let us first examine some important terms: phonological awareness and phoneme acquisition.

Phonological Awareness

Phonological awareness refers to the awareness of and ability to manipulate the phonological segments in words. Specifically, it includes the awareness that words are composed of syllables and phonemes, and that words can rhyme or begin/end with the same sound segment. Phonological awareness enables students to link their knowledge of speech sounds to their knowledge of letters, further enabling them to recognize words in print.

Students who experience difficulty in phonological processing may exhibit some or all of the following problems:

- difficulty with oral expression;
- difficulty with listening comprehension;
- early history of articulation difficulties and/or delayed language;
- difficulty putting sounds together when reading;
- inability to segment spoken words into phonemes and syllables;
- poor reading comprehension due to inability to crack the code; and
- over-reliance on visual memory for word recognition.

Activities

- **Interview the mother of a child with an articulation problem.**
- **With a mirror, observe how you make the common phonemes. Then share your observations with a colleague. Are there differences in how you make the sounds?**

Principles of Phoneme Acquisition

While there is no universally accepted order within which phonemes are acquired, several general conclusions have been offered by researchers regarding the order in which phoneme production occurs (Thomas & Carmack, 1990). In general:

Vowels, acquired before consonants, are usually acquired by age three and are less likely to be misarticulated;

Consonant clusters and blends are not acquired until age seven or eight, although clusters may appear as early as age four.

Manner of articulation refers to *how* a sound is produced. Manner of articulation of consonants follows a certain order of acquisition. **Nasals** (/m/, /n/, /ng/), are acquired first, followed by glides (/w/ /j/), plosives (p, b, t, d, k, g), liquids (l, r), fricatives (/f/, /θ/, /s/, /z/, /ʃ/), and affricates (/tʃ/, /dʒ/).

The following presents a brief definition of the different manners of articulation:

Nasals: Speech sounds with nasal resonance added to them (m, n, and ng).

Glides: Consonant sounds produced while moving from one vowel position to another. Also known as semivowels, these sounds, while clearly consonants, have some vowel-like qualities.

Plosives: Speech sounds produced by building up pressure in the airway and then releasing it; the English sounds /p/, /b/, /k/, and /g/ are plosives.

Liquids: Consonants with vowel-like quality and little air turbulence; also sometimes referred to as semivowels. English /l/ and /r/ are liquids.

Fricatives: A group of consonants produced by constricting the oral cavity and then forcing the air through it; examples include /s/, /z/, and /ʃ/.

Affricates: A group of consonants that have the attributes of both plosives and fricatives that are effectively collapsed into one another; examples include /tʃ/ and /dʒ/.

Place of articulation refers to the place of articulatory contact or constriction. Consonants are acquired in a certain order based on place of articulation. Glottals are acquired first, followed by the labials, velar, alveolar, dentals, and palatals. Sounds are first acquired in the initial position of words. The following represents a brief description of terms associated with places of articulation:

Glottals: Sounds that are produced by keeping the vocal folds open and letting the air pass through. The /h/ sound is an example.

Bilabials: Sounds produced primarily by the two lips. Examples are /p/, /b/, and /m/.

Labiodentals: Sounds produced by the lips and teeth. Examples include /f/ and /v/.

Linguavelars: Sounds produced by the back of the tongue making contact with the soft palate. Examples include the sounds /k/, /g/, and /ng/.

Lingualveolars: Sounds that are produced by raising the tip of the tongue to make contact with the alveolar ridge. The sounds /t/ and /d/ are examples.

Linguadentals: Sounds that are produced by the tongue as it makes contact with the upper teeth. Examples are voiced "th" (/ð/) and unvoiced "th" (/θ/).

Linguapalatals: Sounds that are produced by the tongue as it makes contact with the hard palate. Examples are /ʃ/ and /dʒ/.

There are great individual differences in each child. The age of acquisition for some sounds may vary by as much as three years. It is generally believed that normal acquisition of phonemes continues until approximately seven and a half years of age, but children develop phonemes at various levels. Two of the most frequently used charts in explaining phoneme acquisition are those presented by Templin (1957) and Prather, Hedrick, & Kern (1975). It is generally agreed that professional help should be sought if a child does not correctly pronounce the phonemes by the same relative age as 90 percent of his or her peers. It is important to note that some children take longer to develop their speech to a level where everything can be understood. Research conducted by Prather, Hedrick, and Kern (1975) in the emergence of the correct production of consonants in children aged two to four years provides some averages specific to consonant acquisition. They found that at particular age levels, 90 percent of the children at that age demonstrated normal production of certain consonants in all position within a word:

32 months	n, m, p, t, k
36 months	f, w, b, g, d, j, ŋ
48 months	[s], [t], [d], [z], [f], [r],
Older than 48 months	[l], [r], [z], [dʒ], [ʒ], [θ], [v], [ð]

Sander (1972) was able to predict average age estimates when sounds were acquired and mastered by 90 percent of the children; [ʒ] is one of the last sounds mastered by English-speaking U.S. children, with 90 percent mastery occurring by eight and a half years. Templin (1957) observed that children produce most of the sounds a little later. Bear in mind that there is great variability in the production of speech sounds. The typical ages for mastery of consonant sounds according to Sander (1972) are:

- By age three: /p/, /m/, /h/, /n/, /w/;
- By age four: /b/, /k/, /g/, /d/, /f/, /j/;
- By age six: /t/, /ŋ/, /r/, /l/, and /s/.
- By age seven: /tʃ/, /ʃ/, /dʒ/, /θ/;
- By age eight: /s/, /z/, /v/, and voiced "th" /ð/.
- After the age of eight: /ʒ/.

The International Phonetic Alphabet (IPA)

The sounds of the English language are traditionally indicated by symbols of the International Phonetic Alphabet. The International Phonetic Alphabet is an attempt to present a correspondence between a written symbol and a sound. Each spoken sound is represented by one printed symbol. Because it is impossible to use the traditional alphabet system in recording abnormal articulation errors, the IPA is used. The International Phonetic Alphabet is one of the most recognized sound systems used today. Some advantages are that each written symbol represents one phoneme, and that many of the symbols correspond directly to familiar letters of the alphabet (e.g., p, b, t, d, k, g, m, n, z). One of the disadvantages of this symbol system is that it requires the use of a special font on a keyboard. Table 7.1 presents the IPA symbols and examples of each sound.

TABLE 7.1   *International Phonetic Alphabet (IPA)*

	Symbol	Example	Symbol	Example
Consonants	m	mind	l	live
	n	nose	r	run
	p	pig	ŋ	ring
	h	hand	ʃ	ship
	w	well	tʃ	check
	b	bed	θ	thirst
	k	keep	ð	these
	g	gift	v	vote
	d	date	s	soup
	f	feel	z	zeal
	j	yellow	t	tall
			hw	what
Vowels	i	reef	o	rose
	I	sit	ɔ	wall
	e	face	ɑ	lot
	ɛ	red	ɝ	pert
	aɛ	sat	ʒ	father
	u	food	ə	alert
	ʊ	pull	ʌ	sum
Diphthongs	eɪ	gain	ɔɪ	boy
	oʊ	row	aɪ	kite
	aʊ	town		

Problems of Phonology

Children with phonological problems constitute the largest group of individuals with communication disorders. Voice disorders, deficits in expressive language, and hearing problems occur more frequently in people exhibiting phonological disorders than in individuals without this disorder (Ruscello, St. Louis, & Mason, 1991). Children with phonological disorders may exhibit a significant deficit in speech production perception or in the organization of phonology in comparison to peers (Schwartz, 1994). The severity of this disorder will vary according to the nature and severity of the disability.

Classification of Phonological Errors

Problems in phonology, according to Mercer and Mercer (1989), frequently show up as articulation disorders. The most common problem is that of a child developmentally delayed in phoneme acquisition (articulation). The most frequent types of articulation errors are functional errors: omissions, substitutions, distortions, and additions.

Omission. An articulation error in which a child omits a phoneme at a place that it should occur. For example, the child says "_at" for *cut*. Omissions generally occur in the final position of words, seldom occur in the medial position of words.

Substitution. An articulation error in which a child substitutes or replaces the correct phoneme with a standard or nonstandard phoneme. Examples include *take* for *cake*, in which the phoneme /t/ is substituted for the phoneme ("c") /k/.

Distortion. An approximation of a correct phoneme; the approximation is not accepted as a standard sound. Although the phoneme is visually or acoustically different, it may still retain the basic characteristics of the target phoneme.

Addition. An error in which a child adds a sound. In most cases, the addition error is unstressed [ʌ] after a final consonant. This error is infrequent. An example might be saying "sateʌty" instead of *safety*.

Factors Contributing to Language and Phonological Problems

It is often difficult to pinpoint specifically the cause of an articulation/phonological problem. However, there are some causative factors that may at least contribute to problems of phonology. When children experience difficulty in articulating sounds, it is helpful to identify the factors contributing to the problem. Some of the most common factors include abnormalities of oral–facial structures, other physical handicaps, functional causes, sensory impairments, or a combination of factors (Boone & Plante, 1993).

Other factors may place students "at risk" for language impairment which might place them at risk for language related problems, thus requiring monitoring. The following groups of children have been identified "at risk" or "high risk" for language impairment which subsequently might further place them at risk for language related problems. Included are those from neonatal intensive care units (NICU); diagnosed medical conditions, such as chronic ear infections; biological factors, such as Fetal Alcohol Syndrome (FAS); genetic abnormalities, such as Down Syndrome, neurological anomalies, cerebral palsy; or developmental disorders, such as delayed language.

Chronic Behavior Disorders, Juvenile Delinquency, and Language

Many students with behavioral problems have accompanying speech and language difficulties. (Giddan, 1991). Some reports indicate that as many as sixty-two to ninety-five percent of children being treated for behavioral and emotional problems may also have moderate to severe language problems, ranging from vocabulary to pragmatic deficits (Gallagher, 1999). As a matter of fact, they may be seriously underserved (Casby, 1989). Children labeled as juvenile delinquents have four times more language problems than those in the general population. Further, children exhibiting chronic behavior problems display a higher prevalence of language disorders than in the general population. Areas such as listening vocabulary, speaking vocabulary, speaking grammar, and oral grammar may also be affected. Problems of both comprehension and expression can result in academic problems that can further compound behavioral difficulties.

Mental Retardation and Language Delay

Cognition and language are closely intertwined, so it is no surprise that speech and language problems occur more frequently among people with mental handicaps than in the general population. Articulation problems are the most frequently occurring problems found in people with mental handicaps, followed by delayed language development and restricted or limited active vocabulary (Beirne-Smith, Ittenbach, & Patton, 1998). (A more detailed description of this problem can be found in Chapter 6, Teaching Language Skills to Students with Mild Disabilities.)

"At-Risk" or "High-Risk" Populations for Language Monitoring

The factors that place students "at risk" for language impairment and language-related problems may require monitoring. As mentioned earlier, the following have been identified as "at risk" or "high risk" for language impairment: those from neonatal intensive care units (NICU); those with diagnosed medical conditions, such as chronic ear infections or biological factors, such as Fetal Alcohol Syndrome (FAS); and those with genetic abnormalities, such as Down Syndrome, neurological anomalies, cerebral palsy, or developmental disorders, such as delayed language.

Identifying Children with Language Problems

The classroom teacher plays a vital role in identifying children with possible speech and language difficulties. While a teacher may not have a great deal of background in identifying the problems, it is hoped that this checklist (Owens, 1991) will help you to observe and/or refer youngsters who might benefit from language interventions. Keep in mind that the speech-language professional is available to assist you in learning more about behaviors that might indicate possible language problems.

TABLE 7.2   *Identifying Children with Language Problems*

Directions: The following behaviors may indicate that a child in your classroom has a language impairment that is in need of language intervention. Please check the appropriate items.

_____ Child mispronounces sounds and words.

_____ Child omits words, endings, such as plural -s and past tense -ed.

_____ Child omits small, unemphasized words, such as auxiliary verbs or prepositions.

_____ Child uses an immature vocabulary, overuses empty words, such as 'one' and 'thing,' or seems to have difficulty recalling or finding the right word.

_____ Child had difficulty comprehending new words and concerns.

_____ Child's sentence structure seems immature or over-reliant on forms, such as subject-verb-object. It's unoriginal, dull.

_____ Child has difficulty with one of the following:

_____ Verb tensing	_____ Articles	_____ Auxiliary verbs
_____ Pronouns	_____ Irreg. verbs	_____ Prepositions
_____ Word order	_____ Irreg. plurals	

_____ Child has difficulty relating sequential events.

_____ Child has difficulty following directions.

_____ Child's questions often poorly formed.

_____ Child has difficulty answering questions.

_____ Child's comments often off topic or inappropriate for the conversation.

_____ There are long pauses between a remark and the child's reply or between successive remarks by the child. It's as if the child is searching for a response or is confused.

_____ Child appears to be attending to communication but remembers little of what is said.

Owens, R. E. Jr. (1999). Teacher referral of children with possible language impairment. *Language disorders. A functional approach to assessment and intervention* (3rd ed., p. 373). Boston: Allyn & Bacon.

Assessing Oral Language

Perhaps the single most practical measurement of oral communication competence is intelligibility; therefore, the assessment of intelligibility has important implications. Three major goals for oral language assessment instruments have been outlined by Smith, Finn, and Dowdy (1993) for the classroom teacher and for other people planning intervention for children with problems of phonology. Assessment should determine if a child:

- has functional language in several different environments;
- has functional language with several different groups of people (e.g., peers, parents, teachers, etc.);
- understands reasons for communicating.

Mercer and Mercer (1989) add that the five major reasons for language assessment are to:

- identify children with potential problems in areas of language;
- determine a child's language developmental level;
- plan educational objectives;
- monitor the child's progress; and
- evaluate the language program.

The speech and language pathologist is the person in your school who is trained to diagnose and treat communication problems. If deemed appropriate, a speech-language pathologist, after securing permission from the appropriate people (parents or designated guardian), will schedule a time to evaluate the child's communication skills. Several tests may be used. Some of the formal instruments available to measure oral expression include:

Test of Adolescent & Adult Language (TOAL; Hammill, Brown, Larsen, & Wiederholt, 1990);

Test of Language Development (TOLD; Hammill & Newcomer, 1988);

Clinical Evaluation of Language Fundamentals (CELF; Semel, Wiig, & Secord, 1987);

Goldman-Fristoe Test of Articulation (Goldman & Fristoe, 1986);

Fullerton Language Test for Adolescents (Thorum-Arden, 1975);

Arizona Articulation Proficiency Scale (AAPS) (Fudala & Reynolds, 1986).

Table 7.3 briefly describes each of these measures of oral expression.

Activities
- **Administer a test of oral expression. Share the results.**
- **Interview the parent of a child with phonological problems in your class.**

Strategies for Working with Youngsters Exhibiting Phonological or Articulation Problems

As you have probably already recognized, working with youngsters with communication problems can be a challenge. Your role as the classroom teacher in providing stimulating activities for the child is essential. The following activities are common sense ones, many of which you may be doing already. A speech pathologist remains an excellent reference for sharing additional strategies. Various

TABLE 7.3 *Tests of Oral Expression*

Test of Adolescent and Adult Language, 2 (1987)	**Authors:** Donald Hammill, Virginia Brown, Stephen Larsen, and Lee Wiederholt **Publisher:** Pro-Ed **Ages:** 12–18.6 years + **Purpose:** Provides a norm-referenced measure of language proficiency in adolescent students **Major Areas Assessed:** Receptive and expressive language, both spoken and written **Test Types:** Group, individual, standardized, and norm-referenced
Test of Language Development, Intermediate (1988)	**Authors:** Donald D. Hammill and Phyllis L. Newcomer **Publisher:** Pro-Ed **Ages:** 8.6 through 12.11 **Purpose:** Identifies individuals who are having trouble communicating, diagnoses strengths and weaknesses, evaluates children's progress in prescribed remedial programs, and supports research. **Test Administration:** Raw scores, percentiles, subtests, standard scores, and composite quotients
Clinical Evaluation of Language Fundamentals, Revised (1987)	**Authors:** Eleanor Semel, Elizabeth Wiig, and Wayne Secord **Publisher:** Psychological Corporation **Ages:** 5.16 **Purpose:** Identifies and diagnoses oral language skills in school-age children **Major Areas Assessed:** Receptive and expressive language skills/subtests **Test Types:** Norm scores, total language scores, receptive language score, expressive language score
Goldman-Fristoe Test of Articulation (1986)	**Author:** (s) Ronald Goldman and Macalyne Fristoe **Publisher:** American Guidance Service **Ages:** 2–16+ (individual) **Purpose:** Assesses an individual's ability to articulate the consonant sounds **Major Areas Assessed:** Phonology **Test Scores:** Percentile ranks, norms, reliability, validity
Fullerton Language Test for Adolescents, Revised (1975)	**Author:** R. Thorum-Arden (scoring form and profile) **Publisher:** Consulting Psychologist Press, Inc. **Ages:** 11–18 years **Purpose:** Assesses language and distinguishes normal from impaired language in adolescents **Major Areas Assessed:** 8 subtests **Test Types:** Raw score, mean and standard deviation scores, standard scores
Arizona Articulation Proficiency Scale (1986)	**Authors:** J. Fudala and W. M. Reynolds **Publisher:** Western Psychological Services **Ages:** 1.6 through 13.11 **Purpose:** Assesses each of the American English phonemes, both singly and in clusters, in a variety of contexts **Major Areas Assessed:** Phonology **Test Scores:** Frequency weighting, articulation scores

authors (Meese, 1994; Smith, Finn, & Dowdy, 1993; Gilmore & Norris, 1994) have offered several strategies that might be helpful.

- Model good speaking skills.
- Consistently reinforce children for good listening and for good speaking with peers and teachers.
- Model good listening skills.
- Use concrete activities and experiences for language development.
- Integrate language instruction throughout the school.
- Be sensitive to students' oral language patterns.
- All people who interact with the child should help teach oral language skills, including parents, grandparents, and teachers.
- Read to the child; describe pictures in a book; encourage naming and pointing to familiar objects in the book.
- Never force the child to speak, especially in front of others.
- Recognize and take advantage of the many opportunities available for speech and language learning.
- Coach the child; work actively with the student's oral language skills through role-playing situations, rehearsals, and self-evaluations through videotapes.
- The teacher should model proper speech usage at all times. Record the speech, play the recording back in order for the child to listen to the production. Model the correct speech for the child. This may assist the child in distinguishing proper speech from improper speech.
- Have the child use a mirror in order to watch himself or herself articulating certain words that he or she is having a problem saying. The teacher can assist the student by showing the child the proper manner and place of articulation.
- Read a book to the child and encourage him or her to name and point to familiar objects in the book. Listen for articulation errors and carefully help the child articulate correctly without discouraging the child's desire to read. The goal of this activity is to have the child practice proper speech as much as possible.
- Flashcards are always helpful. Use flashcards and articulate the words on the cards with clear enunciation, then have the child repeat the words.
- Help the child build a lexical base from which he or she can pull labels and categorize and associate new concepts. Field trips can be used to model, expand on, and reinforce the language of experience outside the classroom (Gilmore & Norris, 1994).
- Accept a child's attempts at communication at any age. If you are unable to understand what the child is saying, ask her or him to point to/indicate what is desired.
- For the young child, sound games are fun:
  What does the _____ (animal name) say?
  What does the angry cat (the donkey, the _____) say?
- Follow through on the professional's recommendations.

> ## Activities
>
> * Design and demonstrate a game, for example, "Racing to Be Fire Chief" and "The Word Pond," to develop a selected phoneme.
> * Administer one test of oral expression to a student. Write up and share the results.
> * Interview the parent of a child with a phonological problem. Try to assess the problem in terms of causality, severity, and possible interventions.

Summary

In a generic sense, the term *articulation* refers to the actual movements or joining together of organs. In the act of speaking, multiple organs work together simultaneously in order for sound to be produced. While most people experience little or no difficulty in this most complex act, there are some individuals for whom the act of producing sounds is a challenge.

For the classroom teacher, most of the communication problems that are experienced by some youngsters in the classroom will be problems of articulation: substitutions, omissions, distortions, or additions of sounds. It is hoped that through the information presented in this chapter classroom teachers will have a better understanding of developmental milestones in the communicative process, ways to identify problems of articulation, and strategies that can be employed as a member of the collaborative team in the identification and remediation process. Classroom teachers have an important role, and accurate, applicable, practical, functional knowledge is powerful!

References and Suggested Readings

American Speech-Language-Hearing Association. (1982). Definitions: Communicative disorders and variations. *ASHA, 24,* 949–950.

American Speech-Language-Hearing Association. (1996). *Early identification of speech-language delays and disorders. Let's Talk 32:* Author.

American Speech-Language-Hearing Association. (1996). *Q & A about articulation problems.* Kidsource Online, Inc. [Online]. Available: http://www.healthtouch.com/level1/

Beirne-Smith, M., Ittenbach, R. F., & Patton, J. R. (1998). *Mental retardation* (5th ed.). Upper Saddle River, NJ: Merrill.

Bernstein, D., & Tiegerman, E. (1993). *Language and communication disorders in children* (3rd ed.). New York: Merrill.

Bernthal, J. E., & Bankson, N. W. (1998). *Articulation and phonological disorders.* Boston: Allyn & Bacon.

Bloom, L., & Lahey, M. (1978). *Language development and language disorders.* New York: Wiley.

Boone, D. R., & Plante, E. (1993). *Human communication and its disorders.* Englewood Cliffs, NJ: Prentice-Hall.

Bowen, C. (1999). *Phonological and articulation disorders.* [Online]: Available: http://members.tripod.com/caroline_bowen/phonol_and~artic.htm

Casby, M. W. (1989). National data concerning communication disorders and special education. *Language, Speech, and Hearing Services in the Schools, 20,* 22–30.

Cooter, P. G., Herra, S. A., Logan, C. H., Lyman, D. E., & Morris, D. P. (1997). Phonological awareness and phonetic–graphic conversion: A study of the effects of two intervention paradigms with learning disabled children. Learning disability or learning difference? *Reading Improvement, 71*–89.

Eisenson, J., & Ogilvie, M. (1983). *Communicative disorders in children* (5th ed.). New York: Macmillan.

Fudala, J., & Reynolds, W. M. (1986). *Arizona articulation proficiency scale.* Los Angeles: Western Psychological Services.

Gallagher, T. (1999). Interrelationships among children's language, behavior, and emotional problems. *Topics in Language Disorders, 19,* (2), 1–15.

Giddan, J. (1991). School children with emotional problems and communication deficits: Implications for speech-language pathologists. *Language, Speech, and Hearing Services in the Schools, 22,* 291–295.

Gilmore, S. E., & Norris, G. L. (1994). Using field trips to enhance language treatment. *Language, Speech, and Hearing Services in Schools, 25,* 32–33.

Gleason, J. B. (1993). *The development of language* (3rd ed.). New York: Macmillan.

Goldman, R., & Fristoe, M. (1986). *Goldman-Fristoe test of articulation.* Circle Pines, MN: American Guidance Service.

Gordon-Brannon, M. (1994). Assessing intelligibility. Children's expressive phonologies. *Topics in Language Disorders, 14*(2), 17–25.

Green, R. L. (1994). Speech time is all the time. *TEACHING Exceptional Children, 27*(1), 60–61.

Gustafson, M. (1995). *What to do when you don't understand your child's speech. Communication Skill Builders.* San Antonio, TX: Psychological Corporation.

Hammill, D., Brown, V., Larsen, S., & Wiederholt, L. (1987). *Test of adolescent language, 2.* Austin, TX: Pro-Ed.

Hammill, D., Brown, V., Larsen, S., & Wiederholt, J. (1990). *Test of adolescent and adult language (TOAL-3)* (3rd ed.). Austin, TX: PRO-ED.

Hammill, D., & Newcomer, P. (1988). *Test of language development.* Austin, TX: PRO-ED.

Hulit, L. M., & Howard, M. (1993). *Born to talk: An introduction to speech and language development.* New York: Merrill.

Lowe, R. (1994). Phonology. *Assessment and intervention applications in speech pathology.* Baltimore: Williams & Wilkins.

McReynolds, L. V. (1986). Functional articulation disorders. In G. H. Shames & E. H. Wiig (Eds), *Human communication disorders* (2nd. ed., pp. 445–482). Columbus, OH: Merrill/Macmillan.

Meese, R. L., (1994). *Teaching learners with mild disabilities: Integrating research and practice.* Belmont, CA: Brooks/Cole.

Mercer, C. D., & Mercer, A. R. (1989). *Teaching students with learning problems* (3rd ed.). New York: Macmillan.

National Information Center for Children and Youth with Disabilities. (1996). *General information about speech and language disorders.* NICHCY Fact Sheet Number 11 (FSII): Author.

Owens, R. E., Jr. (1991). *Language development: An introduction* (2nd ed.). Columbus, OH: Merrill.

Owens, R. E., Jr. (1999). *Language disorders. A functional approach to assessment and intervention* (3rd. ed.). Boston: Allyn & Bacon.

Prather, E., Hedrick, D., & Kern, C. (1975). Articulation development in children aged two to four years. *Journal of Speech and Hearing Disorders, 40,* 179–191.

Reed, V. A. (1994). *An introduction to children with language disorders* (2nd ed.). New York: Merrill.

Ruscello, D. M., St. Louis, K. O., & Mason, O. (1991). School-aged children with phonologic disorders: Coexistence with other speech/language disorders. *Journal of Speech and Hearing Research, 34,* 236–42.

Sander, E. K. (1972). When are speech sounds learned? *Journal of Speech and Hearing Disorders, 37,* 55–63.

Schwartz, R. G. (1994). Phonological disorders. In G. H. Shames, E. H. Wiig, & W. A. Secord (Eds.), *Human communication disorders: An introduction* (4th ed., pp. 251–290). New York: Merrill/Macmillan.

Semel, E., Wiig, E., & Secord, W. A. (1987). *Clinical evaluation of language fundamentals.* San Antonio, TX: Psychological Corporation.

Shelton, R. (1995a). *How children acquire speech sounds: Normal, delayed and disordered development.* Communication Skill Builders. San Antonio, TX: Psychological Corporation.

Shelton, R. (1995b). *Types of speech sounds disorders: Articulatory vs. phonologic.* Communication Skill Builders. San Antonio, TX: Psychological Corporation.

Smith, T. E. C., Finn, D. M., & Dowdy, C. A. (1993). *Teaching students with mild disabilities.* Orlando, FL: Harcourt Brace Jovanovich.

Templin, M. C. (1957). *Certain language skills in children: Their development and interrelationships.* Minneapolis: University of Minnesota Press.

Thomas, P., & Carmack, F. (1990). *Speech and language: Detecting and correcting special needs.* Boston: Allyn & Bacon.

Thorum-Arden, R. (1975). *Fullerton language test for adolescents.* Palo Alto, CA: Consulting Psychologists Press.

Van Riper, C., & Erickson, R. (1996). *Speech correction: An introduction to speech pathology and audiology* (9th ed). Boston: Allyn & Bacon.

Vergason, G., & Anderegg, M. L. (1997). *Dictionary of special education and rehabilitation* (4th ed.). Denver, CO: Love Publishing:

Weiss, C. E., & Lillywhite, H. S. (1981). *Communicative disorders: Prevention and early intervention* (2nd ed.). St. Louis: C. V. Mosby.

8

Problems of Voice and Fluency: Identification and Remediation

Martha S. Lue

Objectives

On completion of this section of the chapter, the reader will be able to:

- Define basic terms and concepts relative to voice and voice production;
- Describe basic problems found in adults and school-age children; and
- Describe some basic strategies that the classroom teacher might use in the identification and prevention of some voice problems.

Part I

- Jason, an eight-year-old regular education student, is in the third grade in a local public school. His receptive and expressive language skills are commensurate with his age level as measured by a language screening test. However, in the area of voice, some questions emerged.

    Jason received a medical referral from an otolaryngologist (ENT), who subsequently diagnosed vocal nodules, one of the most common voice problems in children. He has had two evaluations since the initial evaluation and continues to have some hoarseness due to the nodules on his vocal folds. Jason's home life can be described as stable. His parents are very supportive and focus on his accomplishments. Jason's parents help him not to abuse his voice and also to do his breathing exercises. Jason attends speech class for sixty minutes, two days a week. Some of the suggestions offered by the speech-language pathologist were:

- Talk in a quiet voice. No yelling or screaming.
- Have your toys make noises for you. Don't make sound effects such as bombs, motor noises, or animal noises.
- Wave to your friends, instead of yelling at them.
- No whispering. (It irritates vocal nodules.)
- Limit your cheering at ball games.

- The nine-year-old child was referred to the speech-language pathologist because her teacher observed that she constantly lost her voice and was consistently hoarse. Other times, her teacher reported, she sounded very nasal. The speech-language pathologist, with the child's guardian's permission, took the child to see an otolaryngologist to determine if there were structural problems. Tests determined that extra adenoid tissue was interfering with the velopharyngeal port and that she also had some extra tissue on her uvula. The otolaryngologist wanted to do further testing on the child and present the results to the entire diagnostic team for further testing and diagnosis. This process started because of the collaborative effort of the classroom teacher and the speech-language pathologist.

Disorders of Voice

The voice, according to some, represents the window of the soul. It exhibits individual characteristics that are earlier identified by those who know the speaker (Pannbacker & Middleton, 1994). Its uniqueness reflects our own individuality. It is the voice that communicates happiness, sadness, empowerment, strength of character, leadership, stamina, fear, despair, and victory. Voice production has been described as a complicated blend of the respiratory driving force, the highly complex laryngeal muscular interactions, and the placement of the tones in the resonatory system (Stemple, 1996).

The first section of this chapter features basic concepts relative to voice disorders and a description of phonation and the larynx. The disorders of the voice are then placed within the framework of communication. Features of normal and abnormal voices are discussed in relationship to their impact on communication. Finally, strategies that might be used by the classroom teacher in the identification and prevention of possible voice disorders are described.

Phonation and the Larynx

The larynx, commonly referred to as the "voice box," is the chief phonatory organ. Located at the top of the **trachea** (windpipe), it is a complex structure of bone, cartilage, and soft tissue. Without the larynx, phonation in its natural sense does not exist (Sataloff, 1992). As mentioned in Chapter 2, The Speech Process, the larynx serves four major biological protective functions:

- Closing the airway to protect the lungs from food and liquids;
- Impounding the breath, thereby stabilizing the rib cage for more efficient muscle support in lifting;
- Impounding the air for increasing internal abdominal pressure, as in bearing down; and
- Keeping the airway open to allow easy inhalation and exhalation.

The **larynx** also serves a social function, the production of voice for both verbal and nonverbal communication. It contains three distinct regions:

- **Glottis:** Consisting of two bands of tissue known as the true vocal folds. The glottis serves as the opening between the vocal folds;
- **Supraglottis:** A larger area above the true vocal folds that contains several folds of tissue; and the
- **Subglottis:** A small compartment connecting the vocal folds and the windpipe.

Components of the larynx will now be discussed. Included are the vocal folds and the cartilages surrounding the larynx.

Activity

Read the parable, *The Trumpet of the Swan,* by E. B. White (1970). Briefly describe the challenge of not being able to communicate.

Vocal Folds.　When air is exhaled against the **vocal folds,** they vibrate and create sounds, such as /b/, /g/, /d/, and /v/. The greater the air pressure, the louder the sounds. Because the vocal folds in men are usually thicker and longer than in women, they vibrate more slowly, creating a lower pitch or deeper sounding voice.

Cartilages of the Larynx.　The larynx is surrounded by three major cartilages: thyroid, arytenoid, and cricoid. The thyroid cartilage is the largest of the cartilages. The sides of the vocal folds are attached to the wall of the thyroid, and the vocal folds are attached to the arytenoid cartilage, which consists of a pair of small pyramidal cartilages situated in the back of the larynx. The **cricoid** cartilages are ring-shaped cartilages, which lie directly below the thyroid cartilage. The thyroid cartilage forms the foundation or base of the larynx.

Normal Voice/Voice Disorder Defined: In order to determine when a voice is a disorder, let us briefly discuss the term *normal*. Perhaps one of the most salient definitions has been given by Pannbacker & Middleton (1994): A voice is deemed normal if it (1) has an appropriate pitch, for the age, sex, stature, or size of the speaker, (2) is sufficiently loud for the speaking situation, (3) has appropriate oral and nasal **resonance,** and (4) possesses quality that is pleasant to listen to. A voice disorder, on the other hand, is one that affects pitch, loudness, and quality. It calls attention to the speaker on the basis of the speaker's age and cultural expectations. Voice disorders may be the result of faulty structure or function somewhere in the vocal tract in respiration, in phonation, or in resonance (quality) (Boone & McFarlane, 1994). Two general terms used to describe the conditions of one's voice are **aphonia** and **dysphonia.** The term *aphonia* refers to an absence of voice; *dysphonia* refers to an unpleasant voice.

Vocal Problems in Adult Populations

It has been suggested that next to the problem of hearing, voice problems are perhaps the most common type of communication problems found in adults (Boone & Plante, 1993). Problems described in this section include those involving the larynx and the vocal folds.

Debilitating Diseases and Conditions of the Larynx. Several types of debilitating diseases of the larynx have been discussed in the literature. Among them are those due to damage of the muscles by violent shouting, shrieking, screaming, and other brutal abuses of the larynx. Other conditions are associated with

- muscular fatigue from prolonged excessive, though not violent, use;
- excessive load imposed by tumor;
- invasion by neighboring inflammatory conditions; and
- chronic laryngitis caused by abuse.

Activity

Tape-record your voice. Are you surprised at the way it sounds? What were some of your initial reactions?

Tumors and the Larynx. A **tumor** is an abnormal mass of tissue that grows more rapidly than normal and continues to grow after the stimuli that initiated the new growth cease. The tumor can be either benign or malignant. A **benign** (kind) tumor is one that does not form metastases and does not invade and destroy adjacent normal tissue. **Metastasis** is the transfer or spread of a disease from its primary site to a distant location. The most common benign lesion of the larynx is a vocal **polyp** due mainly to vocal abuse. Polyps are usually eliminated through the use of medication and behavior modifications. (Further discussion on vocal polyps is found in a later section of this chapter.) The term *malignant* (evil) tumor is applied to a tumor usually capable of producing metastasis that invades surrounding tissues. Malignant tumors are likely to recur after attempted removal and may cause death of the person unless adequately treated. *Cancer* is the term most frequently used to identify malignant tumors.

Carcinoma of the Larynx.   The term *carcinoma* refers to a cancer that develops from surface tissue. Cancer of the larynx may not become apparent until it produces a change in the voice. A cancer of the larynx may grow rapidly. Treatment includes radiation (use of radium or cobalt rays to destroy cancer cells), surgery, and chemotherapy. When a malignant tumor in the larynx is discovered early, it often can be treated successfully with this radiation, which may leave no or only minimal vocal disorder. Radiation therapy is used for early and small tumors of the larynx. Conservation laryngeal therapy is being used more and holds the potential for minimizing normal tissue destruction, hence preserving the voice (Doyle, 1997).

If surgery is the treatment of choice, part or all of the entire larynx may be removed. Removal of the total larynx is referred to as a *laryngectomy*. People who have had a larynx removed are called **laryngectomees**. When a total laryngectomy is performed, the open end of the trachea is brought to the surface at the base of the neck, where it is attached to an opening in the skin called a *stoma*. The individual then breathes through this opening from the outside directly into the trachea and into the lungs without having the air pass through the nose or mouth. These individuals must develop new modes of communicating, which might include an artificial larynx, learning a substitute voice, or some type of surgical reconstruction. After an individual receives a complete laryngectomy, several options for communicating are available: *electromechanical speech,* **esophageal speech,** and *tracheoesosphageal speech.* In electromechanical speech, a device is placed against the neck and transmits a vibration that produces a voice. With this type of speech, the individual is not frustrated with lack of speech after the operation. A disadvantage is that sometimes the speech sounds very unnatural and machinelike. Esophageal speech uses air that has been pushed into the esophagus to produce sound. The air is pushed back up into the pharynx-esophageal segment to create resonance. The speech produced is more natural sounding and there is no electric device to use. A disadvantage is that the success rate is low; 25 to 30 percent of people are able to use this method because it is very difficult. The speech is so low-pitched that it is often hard to understand what the person is saying.

Tracheoesophageal speech is a process in which the tracheoesophageal puncture (TEP) is surgically placed in the site where the laryngectomy occurred. It involves a silicon voice prosthesis. Advantages include a much more natural sounding voice than the other methods do and the success rate is very high. Daily maintenance is required. A recurrent leakage at the site has sometimes been reported. Over time, the method is costly.

Trauma and Surgical Modifications of the Larynx. There are basically three degrees of trauma and surgical modifications that may occur: cord repair, cordectomy (removal of one vocal fold), or complete removal of the larynx itself. In some cases, if the cartilages of the larynx are injured, they may heal in such a way that normal motion is not possible.

Conditions of the Vocal Folds

Conditions of the vocal folds that might cause voice problems are classified as **psychogenic** (functional) problems or **organic factors** (a problem with a physical cause). Psychogenic problems may be related to stress and/or anxiety. There are three kinds of **functional dysphonia:** (1) The vocal folds vibrate without a closed phase or in a lax manner (breathiness); (2) The vocal folds are squeezed together so tightly that the folds cannot vibrate normally (producing qualities of harshness or tightness); (3) *tension-fatigue syndrome* is characterized by abnormal pitching of the voice and poor breath stream control (Kaufman & Blalock, 1988). These conditions are referred to as *functional dysphonia* because they do not result from an organic pathology (Boone & McFarlane, 1994). Problems related to organic factors (having a physical cause) may include, but are not limited to, **paralysis,** a condition in which the vocal folds do not abduct or adduct, and **ankylosis,** an impairment of the arytenoid movement caused by cancer, arthritis, and so on of the arytenoid cartilage (situated in the back of the larynx).

Carcinoma of the Vocal Folds. A carcinoma can grow on one or both vocal folds, and subsequently affect their vibration. Oftentimes these are rapidly growing tumors and do not become evident until there is a change in voice or similar problems, such as a persistent sore throat. If such occurs, a physician should be consulted immediately.

Vocal Nodules or Vocal Polyps? Sometimes doctors identify vocal problems that interfere with speaking, making **abduction** and **adduction** of the vocal cords difficult. Two of the most commonplace are vocal nodules and vocal polyps. Both are commonplace among rock singers, cheerleaders, and people who talk in a sharp or strained voice (Dickey, 1994). Often the terms *nodules* and *polyps* are used to label structural abnormalities; many times there is confusion when these terms are used interchangeably. There is a difference between vocal nodules and vocal polyps. Although both may be initially noncancerous, professional attention is needed for specific identification and treatment. Having **vocal nodules** is like having a callus on a toe. There is a callus buildup of tissue on the vocal fold. Vocal nodules can occur on one (unilateral) or both (bilateral) vocal folds. While vocal rest usually clears the nodules, prolonged abuse of the folds may result in larger and more persistent nodules. A **vocal polyp** is similar to having an ulcer on some part of the body. The polyp is usually filled with fluid or other organic matter. Polyps are softer than nodules and are typically unilateral. Polyps may also occur in other parts of the body such as the nose, respiratory tract, and digestive tract.

Reflection

Your friend, who is now a sophomore in college, has been cheerleading for about eight years. She now complains about being chronically hoarse, especially early in the morning. What suggestions/recommendations can you offer her?

Voice Disorders in School-Age Children

It is imperative to note that if you suspect that a child does have a voice problem, the speech-language pathologist should be consulted and the parents urged to get medical help immediately (Davis & Harris, 1992). In this section, common problems of pitch, loudness, and quality that affect school-age children will be described.

Problems of Pitch

A child's pitch may be too high or low for her or his age or sex with respect to cultural expectations. Pitch discrepancies may be a result of either organic or functional causes. Examples of causes may vary from vocal abuse (screaming/yelling) or edema to cerebral palsy and vocal nodules.

Optimum pitch is that pitch level at which an individual is able to vocalize most efficiently. This is the level at which good quality, loudness, and ease of production are found.

Monotone pitch refers to pitch that lacks variation, emotional affect, and little change or flexibility. It exhibits little energy or enthusiasm. It may also be related to the presence of a hearing loss or emotional or personality factors. To avoid or eliminate a monotone pitch, one is encouraged to find the optimum pitch.

To find your own speaking pitch range:

- With the musical scale in mind, intone the vowel /a/ at your lowest pitch level.
- Go up the scale a level at a time until you reach falsetto.
- Repeat, using the sound /m/.
- The two levels should match. If not, take the wider range.

Within a pitch range, the optimal pitch is about the third or fourth level from your lowest pitch. Thus, if one can intone twelve levels, optimal pitch is at about level three or four. An acceptable range for a normal, healthy voice is about one octave, for example, the notes lower **C** to high **C.**

Problems of Intensity (Loudness)

Intensity refers to the loudness of one's voice. Optimal loudness is one that is appropriate to the situation and numbers of listeners (Pannbacker & Middleton, 1994). Problems of intensity may include a voice that is either too soft or too loud to be effectively heard. Too loud or too soft characteristics might include an unpleasant, piercing voice or conversational volume louder/softer than other speakers and speech volume inappropriate for the situation. Excessive volume may contribute to the formation of nodules or polyps on the vocal folds (Thomas & Carmack, 1990). An immediate symptom and warning to modify vocal behavior is laryngitis. In a typical conversational setting, a voice that is too soft would be less than 50 dB, whereas one that is too loud would exceed 85 dB. The size of the room, the audience, and the purpose of the speaker should determine the vocal volume.

Problems of Quality

Problems of quality include voices that are described as hoarse, nasal, or breathy. The earliest warning sign of pathology of the larynx is hoarseness. Because of the potential seriousness, it is extremely important to seek and obtain medical clearance before trying any strategies with the child. Early indicators of problems of quality include: chronic hoarseness, reduced vocal range, repeated loss of voice, frequent laryngitis, some inaudible speech sounds, or difficulties making oral responses in class (Thomas & Carmack, 1990).

Nasality is associated with a relaxed soft palate during the act of vocalization. If there is generally sluggish soft palate action, speech is likely to sound nasal. Children who have had their adenoids removed frequently change from having markedly denasal voices to having characteristically nasal voices. When enlarged adenoids are present, a child needs to elevate the soft palate very little to result in obstructing the opening of the nasal cavity. After the removal of the adenoidal tissue, the habit of partial elevation of the soft palate may persist, and nasality may then occur during the production of all speech sounds.

Two types of nasal voice are frequently noted in the literature: **hypernasality** and **hyponasality.** In hypernasality, the voice sounds as if it were coming through the nose. This condition occurs when there is excessive nasal resonance, airflow, and sound-wave transmission through the nose. Children who have cleft palate are often hypernasal, as are individuals who are deaf. Hyponasality, sometimes referred to as *denasality,* occurs when there is insufficient nasal resonance. In this condition, people sound as if they have a severe allergy, head cold, or stopped up nose. It is usually caused by some kind of structural blockage that prevents the flow of air and sound waves from passing through the nose. In this condition, there is insufficient nasal resonance for the three nasal phonemes /m/, /n/, and /ng/, and nearly total lack of nasal resonance for vowels.

The child who exhibits a breathy voice may have difficulty being heard. Students who exhibit excessive breathiness when speaking may produce weak speech volume, and inhale frequently. This breathiness could result from misuse of the voice or as a result of pathological problems (e.g., cancer).

Still another classification of disorder of quality has been described by Stemple (1996), the medically fragile child. This child has voice disorders as a result of congenital, developmental, or acquired disorders, and may have cerebral palsy, cystic fibrosis, or other respiratory or chronic health impairments.

Vocal Hygiene and the Classroom Teacher

Vocal behaviors for many careers place members at risk for developing a vocal pathology (Long, Williford, Olson, & Wolfe, 1998; Smith, Hoffman, Kirchner, Lemke, & Taylor, 1998). Principles for maintaining good vocal hygiene are important for the teacher who must remain "voiced" (Martin, 1994; Kereiakes, 1996). These same techniques and principles may be used in working with children in the classroom. Proper vocal hygiene includes developing healthy attitudes about the use and treatment of the vocal mechanism (Rosen, 1998). To prevent vocal problems in children, Pindzola (1993) has suggested vocal hygiene programs, including an explanation of the process of voice production, and a description of the anatomy and physiology of the vocal folds, especially in relationship to inflammation or growth. Other strategies have been suggested as well.

- **Keep the Yelling Down**
  A major cause of vocal abuse leading to damage of the vocal folds is excessive shouting or cheering. It's not a coincidence that cheerleaders have so many voice problems. Teachers are reported to be at a higher risk of voice problems than the general population, and females are twice as likely as males to report voice problems (Russell, Oates, & Greenwood, 1997). People who teach physical education are more prone to experience a voice problem than any other teaching discipline (Smith, Hoffman, Kirchner, Lemke, & Taylor, 1998).

- **Get Breath Support from the Stomach**
  If you must talk loudly, use your stomach muscles to punch out more air. Avoid tensing the neck and upper chest area because that constricts the larynx. Actors and skilled public speakers know that, as with toothpaste, you get better results if you squeeze from the bottom of the tube. Dickey (1994) further suggests practicing diaphragmatic breathing, breathing from deep down in the small of one's back, as when lying on one's back. As one inhales, one should feel the back expand and the stomach pushing out. This allows the speaker to project the voice without hurting it.

- **Be Wary of Noisy Places**
  Trying to talk for any length of time in a noisy area can be very hard on your voice. It might be wiser in such situations to spend more time listening, find a form of nonverbal communication, or retire to a quiet place.

- **Cough Carefully**
  Avoid vigorous coughing and throat-clearing as much as possible. It is suggested that clearing the throat, in the absence of illness, more than ten times an hour is too much. Drinking eight to ten glasses of water a day to keep the throat moist is also recommended.

- **Easy Does It**
  Avoid taking a deep breath and then initiating a sound with a sudden, abrupt release. Use an easy onset by bringing the vocal cords together at the same instant you release air.

- **Natural Is Best**
  Use the pitch level that is natural for you. Many people damage their vocal folds by trying to assume the low-pitched voice of authority.

- **Silence Is Cold**
  Try to limit the amount of talking when you have a cold. When vocal folds are swollen, they can be damaged easily by just normal opening and closing movements.

- **Guard against Inhalants**
  Research suggests that tobacco smoke may be one of the most toxic substances one can inhale. Also, guard against breathing aerosol products, taking precaution to wear a mask in dusty environments.

- **Tape-Record Yourself**
  Use a tape recorder in normal conversation. When you play it back, pay attention to your breathing. Learn to breathe often enough so that your voice production is smooth.

- **Keep Cool**
  Remember that stress is reflected in body tension. Keep in touch with your level of tension and learn to relax.

- **Early Detection Is Important**
  Some of the warning signs of possible vocal abuse are an unsteady pitch level, pitch breaks, hoarseness (lasting more than three weeks), and a voice that fatigues easily. These and other dramatic vocal changes need to be reported to a doctor; seek medical attention immediately. Get a thorough laryngeal examination so that a more serious problem will be prevented from developing. Get good advice about vocal hygiene from a speech-language pathologist. If a voice deviation is present also, have a child's hearing checked. Talk with appropriate loudness or pitch levels and encourage the child to do the same. If laryngitis is present, limit the amount of talking the child does. Be especially careful in considering removal of the adenoids (get a second opinion). Seek early surgical or other medical treatment only when organic conditions are present such as cysts, tumors, and diseases of the vocal folds. Refer a child to a speech-language pathologist if the child's voice calls attention to itself, such as when sounds seem nasal, speech sounds monotonous, or there are excessive pitch breaks.

Summary

This section of the chapter provides important information for the classroom teacher and for those professionals in need of a sustained voice (actors, ministers, etc.). The voice is a uniquely complex instrument. There is much to learn about how it works and all of the many possible things that can go wrong. Most of us have experienced temporary vocal dysfunctioning, such as laryngitis or problems related to allergies that affect the quality, loudness, and pitch of our voice. While temporary in nature, these conditions show us how wonderful, yet sensitive, this vocal apparatus is. Disorders of voice—problems involving pitch, loudness, and quality—affect individuals of all ages, from the young child who screams too much and too loudly to the individual who has had to have the larynx removed because of a malignancy. Guard your voice with care. Model appropriate vocal behavior, and chances are your students will try to do the same.

Part II

Problems of Fluency

Objectives

On completion of this section of the chapter, the reader will be able to describe:

- Some problems of fluency and their causes in school-age children; and,
- Some strategies that the classroom teacher might use in the prevention and remediation of these problems.

- Nine-year-old Jonathan, one of three children, cannot remember a time when he did not stutter. (Jonathan's father also stutters.) He finds himself dysfluent when he has to read out loud and recite in front of his classmates. He wants to be in his class's end-of-the-year school play, but does not like speaking in front of groups. Jonathan receives individual speech therapy, twice a week, thirty minutes each day, from the speech-language pathologist at his school. He is very bright and is on the school's honor roll.

- The twenty-year-old college student with a slight stuttering problem is an elementary education major. He speaks English as a second language. His first spoken language is French Creole. He becomes very dysfluent when speaking to adults that he does not know, when he is trying to talk at a fast pace, when he is excited, and when he is using complex expressive vocabulary. When speaking with people of his same age group, he has minimal problems. The major problem that he exhibits when stuttering is hesitation.

The process of communication separates human beings from other species. These vignettes indicate the struggle that some speakers have in trying to communicate verbally. Difficulty communicating with other human beings is obviously a very serious problem that can affect all aspects of a child's school or home life. Teachers as well as family members must show responsibility in seeking and applying methods for helping the child who has such difficulty.

Generally, all children experience dysfluencies from time to time. Young children, in particular, are in a period of rapid language and speech development. Dysfluencies may be normal and should be expected as children attempt to assimilate their growing linguistic awareness into their speech patterns (Swan, 1993). For a small number of children, however, the dysfluencies intensify and become problematic to the speaker as well as to the listener. This section of the chapter will explore two of the most common problems of fluency: **stuttering** and **cluttering**. Strategies that the classroom teacher might use in the identification, prevention, and remediation of these problems will also be addressed.

Components of Speech Flow

In order for individuals to communicate effectively, the following components of speech flow must be present:

- rhythm: the timing of speech units;
- rate: the speed with which units are produced;
- fluency: the smoothness with which units of speech flow together.

ASHA (1999) describes fluency as "the aspect of speech production that refers to the continuity, smoothness, rate, and/or effort with which phonologic, lexical, morphologic, and/or syntactic language units are spoken" (p. 30). As described in Chapter 3, Early Communication Development, during the preschool years speech and language skills of children develop rapidly. Bloodstein (1987) argues that this is usually the period when stuttering begins. It is plausible to state, then, that fluency problems occur when there are disruptions in the rhythm, rate, and fluency for the speaker. The term *dysfluency* refers to "breaks in the continuity of producing phonologic, lexical, morphologic, and/or syntactic language units in oral speech" (ASHA, 1999, p. 30).

> *Activity*
>
> **Interview a person who stutters. Invite him or her to speak to your class.**

Descriptions of Stuttering

It is believed that approximately 3 million people in the United States stutter. The vast majority of individuals begin to stutter between the ages of two and six; the mean age of onset is five years (Lablance, Steckol, & Smith, 1994).

While no clear-cut definition of stuttering has emerged, most researchers view the disorder as a fluency problem that may include repetitions, prolongations, hesitations, and interjections (Shames & Rubin, 1986; Perkins, 1990; Cooper, 1997). The dysfluencies most often occur on specific sounds and syllables. Other descriptions include one offered by Meltzer (1992), who concluded that stuttering is a disruption in the rhythm of speech as a result of abnormalities in the timing and movement of muscles in the respiratory, laryngeal, and peripheral organs of articulation. These disruptions usually occur frequently and are marked in character and are not readily controllable by the speaker (Perkins, 1992).

Van Riper (1982) suggests that when the forward flow of speech is interrupted by a motorically disrupted sound, syllable, or word by the speaker's reaction to his or her environment or any kind of stimulus, stuttering occurs. Bloodstein (1987) further suggests that stuttering develops out of normal-sounding dysfluency, but not because of misdiagnosis. Instead, stuttering develops when speech and fragmentation become magnified by communicative pressure.

> *Activity*
>
> **Find information on Jacobsen's Relaxation Therapy or another progressive relaxation citation. Cite specific implications for the dysfluent individual.**

Normal Dysfluency and Stuttering

Perkins (1990) has identified five temporal elements of speech flow. Problems can occur when one or more of these elements are compromised. Some disruptions are sometimes observed in both normal speakers and in people who stutter.

- Sequence: the order of speech sounds necessary for meaning not to be compromised;
- Duration: the length of time that any phonetic element lasts;
- Rate: the speed with which phonetic elements of various durations are articulated together;
- Rhythm: the phonetic patterns of a language when spoken with a flowing continuity; and
- Fluency: the smooth pattern with which sounds are articulated together.

The speech of someone who stutters may be characterized by duration changes and rate and rhythm alterations with frequent interruptions of smooth fluency between one sound and another.

Activity

Identify four myths regarding the cause or onset of stuttering.

Perspectives on Stuttering

Just as there are varying definitions of stuttering, there are different perspectives and approaches to therapy for the disorder. Listed are but a few of the perspectives that have been reported in the literature:

- Stuttering appears to be a multidimensional problem including emotional, behavioral, interpersonal, and social factors;
- It involves linguistic, cognitive, and psychological variables (Shames & Rubin, 1986);
- Stuttering appears to have a genetic basis (Yairi, 1998). Children of people who stutter are more likely than other children to stutter even when the parent stopped stuttering long before the child was born;
- Stuttering occurs more frequently in males than in females and is found in a large variety of cultures and languages;
- It tends to be more common, to endure for more years, in boys compared to girls;
- Children who stutter find it difficult to coordinate respiration, the functioning of the larynx, and articulation. The timing of these sets of behavior, so necessary for normal speech, may be different than in the normal population;
- Stuttering becomes an increasingly formidable problem in the teen years as dating and social interaction begins; and
- Often speech and language disorders coexist in people who stutter.

Other observations about stuttering suggest that about 80 percent of those who have stuttered at one time or the other spontaneously recover from it. Yairi (1998) also noted that a single, specific gene may cause stuttering, and its effect may lessen and even disappear over time. The longer stuttering persists in any given person, the more likely it is that associated emotional problems will develop. No one who stutters, regardless of the severity of dysfluency, stutters at all times. Almost all people who stutter have times when their speech is relatively, if not completely, free of significant hesitations, blocks, repetitions, or prolongations.

People who stutter often respond to their problems by avoiding talking or avoiding social interactions where talking is expected, and they may respond to the problem by being overly aggressive. They may elicit negative reactions in listeners from their aggression as well as their stuttering.

has yet to be proven

Activity

Compare and contrast three theories on the causation of stuttering

Prevalence

Stuttering is thought to affect approximately 1 percent of the population world-wide. Prevalence figures in the United States, however, vary from this "norm," where figures range from .03 to 2.1 percent in school-age children. Bloodstein (1987) notes, for example, that in countries other than the United States, there are also tremendous discrepancies. In the Czech Republic and Slovakia, for example, the figure is 4.7 percent.

Ninety-eight percent of cases of stuttering begin before age ten (Mahr & Leith, 1992). Research suggests that 25 percent of all children go through a stage of development during which they stutter, and 4 percent may stutter for six months or more.

Activity

Develop three strategies that you, as a teacher, have found or might find effective in working with dysfluent speakers. Compare and contrast the terms *stuttering* and *cluttering*, and cite specific examples of each.

Research Related to Stuttering

Stuttering and Family Intervention

Mallard (1998) described a program designed to assist families in managing stuttering problems. The two-week program, involving elementary age children who stutter, is family oriented, and includes siblings. The rationale for this involvement, as described by Mallard, is that if the family is the focus of treatment, "taking into account the culture and communication patterns within the family, then the child who stutters will have assistance as needed from those who understood the child best" (p. 127). The program focuses on speech therapy, social skills, and transfer activities—all combined in problem-solving. This method further encourages children to attempt to solve their problems in their own way. The speech-language pathologist assists the family in finding the most appropriate technique for accomplishing this. Results indicated that 82 percent of the children did not need further therapy for stuttering at the end of the program. Though the findings did not necessarily mean they no longer stuttered, it did mean that they had learned how to manage their stuttering without further assistance from a professional.

In a study of 169 adult and adolescent people who stutter, Poulos and Webster (1991) noted that 112 had family members who stuttered. Of the ones who did not, many had childhood traumas that induced stuttering. When asked about family history, including language problems other than stuttering as well as any traumas that could have started the stuttering, the results indicated that almost two-thirds of the people who stuttered had family members who stuttered. All of the family members were lifetime stutterers.

Anxiety.   In the development of speech fluency, anxiety appears to play a major role. Craig (1990) reported the result of a study of 120 people who stutter, most of whom were men. They were tested on state and trait anxiety before and after behavior therapy. The anxiety levels were compared to those of nonstutterers of the same sex and occupations. The results showed that those who stuttered had higher fear levels and more chronic anxiety than the nonstutterers. After treatment, however, the trait anxiety level (chronic) was at a normal level.

Activity

Review three different children's books in which one of the characters stuttered. Compare and contrast the speaking behaviors of each of the characters.

Stuttering and Special Groups.   Stuttering appears to be related to other mental handicapping conditions. The occurrence of stuttering in individuals with mental disabilities varies from 0.8 percent to 20.3 percent. In minority populations, however, the types of dysfluencies are similar to those in other populations (Lilies, Legman, Christensen, & St. Ledger, 1992).

Parental Influence.   The way in which some parents talk may have some influence on a child who stutters. Chollar (1988) reports that while some stuttering may be due to genetic disorders, it could also be exacerbated by the modeling of undesirable speech behaviors of the child's parents. For example, speaking too rapidly in long complex utterances, with sophisticated vocabulary, may not be a good model for a three-year-old.

Reflection

It has been suggested that all people are dysfluent at one time or the other. Cite three instances when you were dysfluent.

Description of Cluttering

Cluttering, as defined by ASHA (1999), is a fluency disorder characterized by a rapid and/or irregular speaking rate, excessive dysfluencies, and often other symptoms, such as language or phonological errors and attention deficits. Gitlin & Daly (1994) add that some individuals who clutter do not speak faster than their peers, but instead speak too fast for their own oral coordination abilities.

Cluttering is characterized by the clutterer's unawareness of her or his disorder, by a short attention span, by disturbances in perception, articulation, formulation of speech, and often by excessive speed of delivery, and the speech is often so rapid as to be unintelligible. The speaker may clip off speech sounds. ASHA (1999) further defines cluttering as "a constellation of symptoms, including fluency problems" (p. 35). There also appears to be a strong correlation between cluttering, learning disabilities, and ADHD.

Thomas and Carmack (1990) note that early cluttering of speech may lead to stuttering behavior later, and that both cluttering and stuttering behaviors may occur in the same speaker in as many as 40 percent of the cases. Moreover, one of the more noticeable distinctions between people who clutter and those who stutter is that oftentimes the individual who clutters is not aware that a communicative problem exists. In some cases, people who clutter may be attempting to speak faster than their systems can handle (Lees, Boyle, & Woolfson, 1996).

Activity

Prepare a short annotated bibliography on research related to stuttering.

Therapy

While there is not consistent agreement on the best therapy approaches for individuals who clutter, research suggests that the first step in the treatment by the speech-language pathologist may be that of convincing the individual that a serious problem exists and that therapy is indeed warranted.

St. Louis and Myers (1998) suggest using the analogy of a speedometer in which "rapid speech is above the 'speed limit' and 'speed tickets' are given for exceeding the 'limit.' " Because many people who clutter may have limited awareness of their rapid and irregular speech rate, St. Louis and Myers suggest that it might be helpful if these individuals are directed to count silently with their fingers or raise and lower their forearm to coincide with pauses. Other efforts toward remediation include: assisting the person who clutters in becoming aware of her or his speech and assuming more responsibility for successful communication to others (Thomas & Carmack, 1990); developing relaxation techniques; using positive self-talk and delayed auditory feedback techniques (Gitlin & Daly, 1994).

Activity

Survey several teachers in the local school district. Ask them if they have had dysfluent speakers in the classroom, and what strategies they've employed in working with the student.

Disorders of Fluency: Helpful Hints for Prevention/Remediation

As a classroom teacher, it is your role to present a communication environment that is nurturing and conducive for all learners. The following strategies will be helpful in this discussion.

- Find quiet time during the day to share language with the child; pull away from anything that is distracting.
- Have students read aloud in unison in a small group. Gradually reduce the size of the group until the child is reading one-on-one with a naturally slow reader. The speaker who is assisting the person who stutters should lower her or his voice and eventually say every other word. This is known as the "adaptation effect" as described by Schwartz (1976).

When communicating with a person who stutters, The Stuttering Foundation of America (1999) offers these tips:

- Ignore the temptation to finish sentences or fill in words for people who stutter. Don't say, "slow down," "take a deep breath," "relax." Such advice is not helpful.
- Maintain eye contact and wait patiently until the person is finished.
- Talk in a relaxed, but slower than normal manner.
- Be patient on the telephone. People who stutter have more trouble controlling their speech when they are talking on the phone than in a face-to-face situation.

Weiss and Lillywhite (1981) also suggest:

- As a listener, do not react emotionally when a child is having difficulty with fluency.
- Do not interrupt or say the word for the child when the child is trying to say something.
- Be a good listener; this requires considerable effort.

- Never force the child to talk or perform orally.
- Have reasonable expectations for the child; do not expect too much too soon.
- Early counseling with a speech-language pathologist is indispensable.

In addition, Swan (1993) suggests:

- Give all children your full attention when engaging them in conversation, especially the child who stutters.
- Create a relaxed unhurried learning environment. Use and model a relaxed, unhurried rate of speech for all students.
- Demonstrate and encourage polite speaking manners; do not allow students to interrupt, speak for others, or finish their words for them.
- Provide successful group speaking experiences for all children, such as choral speaking, reading, and singing.

Reflection

- **Evaluate your own speech in terms of fluency. Write a brief description of it.**
- **Develop your own theory regarding stuttering. Be ready to share it with a peer.**

Stuttering at a Glance: Things Teachers Should Know

- Stuttering affects an estimated 1.5 to 3.5 million Americans, half of whom are young children.
- Stuttering affects four times as many males as females.
- While three-fourths of the children who stutter will spontaneously recover from it, the remaining one-fourth do not and only recover after minimal or time-consuming therapy.
- Early detection of stuttering can lead to appropriate treatment and increase the likelihood of full recovery for many children.
- Dysfluencies are normal and are to be expected as children attempt to assimilate their growing linguistic awareness.
- Although stuttering is a communication problem, there is an accompanying emotional aspect to the problem.
- The Stuttering Foundation of America maintains an Internet site at http://www.stuttersfa.org and a toll-free number at 1-800-992-9392.

Summary

In this section of the chapter, problems of fluency were discussed. Two of the most common types of fluency problems, stuttering and cluttering, were described. Identification, remediation, and prevention strategies were highlighted. As a classroom teacher, your role will be multifaceted: identifying and referring the child suspected of having a problem, following through on strategies provided by the speech-language pathologist, and developing and maintaining a communicative environment that is nurturing, supportive, and encouraging.

References and Suggested Readings

Ambrose, N., Yairi, E. & Cox, N. (1993). Genetic aspects of early childhood stuttering. *Journal of Speech & Hearing Research, 36,* 701–706.

American Speech-Language-Hearing Association Special Interest Division 4: Fluency and Fluency Disorders (1999, March). Terminology pertaining to fluency and fluency disorders: Guidelines. *ASHA, 41* (Suppl. 19), 29–36.

Aronson, A. E. (1985). *Clinical voice disorders* (2nd ed.). New York: Thieme-Stratton.

Bloodstein, O. (1984). Speech pathology and speech disorders. In O. Bloodstein (Ed.), *Speech pathology: An introduction* (2nd ed., pp. 1–5). Boston: Houghton Mifflin.

Bloodstein, O. (1987). *A handbook on stuttering* (4th ed.). Chicago: National Easter Seal Society.

Boone, D., & McFarlane, S. C. (1994). *The voice and voice therapy* (5th ed.) Englewood Cliffs, NJ: Prentice-Hall.

Boone, D., & Plante, E. (1993). Disorders of communication in adults. In D. Boone & E. Plante (Eds.), *Human communication and its disorders* (2nd ed, pp. 135–162.). Englewood Cliffs, NJ: Prentice-Hall.

Chollar, S. (1988, December). Stuttering: The parental influence. *Psychology Today, 22,* (12), 12–17.

Cooper, E. B. (1986). Treatment of dysfluency: Future trends. *Journal of Fluency Disorders, 11,* 317–327.

Cooper, E. B. (1997). Stuttering: A short history of the disorder. *Journal of Fluency Disorders, 24,* (3), 73–76.

Craig, A. (1990). An investigation into the relationship between anxiety and stuttering. *Journal of Speech and Hearing Disorders, 55,* 290–294.

Davis, C. N., & Harris, T. B. (1992). Teachers' ability to accurately identify disordered voices. *Language, Speech, and Hearing Services in Schools, 23,* 136–140.

Dickey, M. (1994, December). Finding your voice. *Washingtonian, 30,* 45–49.

Doyle, P. (1997). Voice refinement following conservation is urgent for cancer of the larynx: A conceptual framework for treatment intervention. *American Journal of Speech-Language Pathology, 6,* 27–35.

Gitlin, D., & Daly, D. (1994). Speech cluttering. *Journal of the American Medical Association, 272,* (7), 565.

Hedge, M. N. (1995). *Introduction to communicative disorders* (2nd ed.). Austin, TX: PRO-ED.

Kaufman, J. A. (1998). What are voice disorders and who gets them? Center for voice disorders of Wake Forest University [On-line]. Available: http://www.bgsm.edu/voice_disorders.html

Kaufman, J. A., & Blalock, P. (1988). Vocal fatigue and dysphonia in the professional voice user: Bogart-Bacall syndrome. *Laryngoscope, 98,* 493–498.

Kereiakes, T. J. (1996). Clinical evaluations and treatment of vocal disorders. *Language, Speech, and Hearing Services in Schools, 27,* 240–243.

LaBlance, G. R., Steckol, K. F., & Smith, V. L. (1994). Stuttering: The role of the classroom teacher. *TEACHING Exceptional Children, 27,* 10–12.

Lees, M., Boyle, B. E., & Woolfson, L. (1996). Is cluttering a motor disorder? *Journal of Fluency Disorders, 21,* 281–287.

Lilies, B. Z., Legman, J., Christensen, L., & St. Ledger, J. (1992). A case description of verbal and signed disfluencies of a 10 year old boy who is retarded. *Language, Speech, and Hearing Services in Schools, 23,* (2), 107–112.

Long, J., Williford, H., Olson, M. S., & Wolfe, V. (1998). Voice problems and risk factors among aerobics instructors. *Journal of Voice, 12,* (2), 197–207.

Mahr, G., & Leith, W. (1992). Psychogenic stuttering of adult onset. *Journal of Speech & Hearing Research, 35,* 283–286.

Mallard, A. R. (1998). Using problem solving procedures in family management of stuttering. *Journal of Fluency Disorders, 23,* 127–135.

Mallard, A. R., & Westbrook, J. (1988). Variables affecting stuttering therapy in school settings. *Language, Speech and Hearing Services in Schools, 19,* 362–370.

Martin, S. (1994). Voice care and development for teachers: Survey report, *Voice,* 92–98.

Meltzer, A. (1992). Horn stuttering. *Journal of Fluency Disorders, 17,* 257–264.

Moore, G. P., & Hicks, D. M. (1994). Voice disorders. In G. H. Shames, E. A. Wiig, & W. A. Secord. (Eds.), *Human communication disorders: An introduction* (4th ed., pp. 292–335). New York: Merrill/Macmillan.

Nippold, M. A. (1990). Concomitant speech and language disorders in stuttering children: A critique of the literature. *Journal of Speech & Hearing Disorders, 55,* 51–60.

Pannbacker, M., & Middleton, G. (1994). Voice disorders. In S. Adler & D. King, *Oral communication problems in children and adolescents* (2nd ed., pp. 103–119). Boston: Allyn & Bacon.

Perkins, W. H. (1990). *The nature of stuttering.* Englewood Cliffs, NJ: Prentice-Hall.

Perkins, W. H. (1992). *Stuttering prevented.* San Diego, CA: Singular.

Pindzola, R. (1993). Clinical exchange: Materials for use in vocal hygiene programs for children. *Language, Speech and Hearing Services in Schools, 24,* 174–176.

Poulos, M. G., & Webster, W. G. (1991). Family history as a basis for subgrouping people who stutter. *Journal of Speech & Hearing Research, 34,* 5–10.

Rosen, C. A. (1998). Evaluating hoarseness: Keeping your patient's voice healthy. *American Family Physician, 57,* (11), 2775–2783.

Russell, A., Oates, J., & Greenwood, K. M. (1997). Prevalence of voice problems in teachers. *Journal of Voice, 12,* (4), 467–479.

Ryan, B. P. (1992). Articulation, language, rate, & fluency characteristics of stuttering and nonstut- tering preschool children. *Journal of Speech and Hearing Research, 35,* 333–342.

Sataloff, R. T. (1992). The human voice. *Scientific American, 267,* 110–111.

Schwartz, M. (1976). *Stuttering solved.* Philadelphia: Lipincott.

Shames, G. H., & Rubin, H. (1986). *Stuttering then and now.* New York: Merrill/Macmillan.

Smith, E., Hoffman, H., Kirchner, H. L., Lemke, J. H., & Taylor, M. (1998). Voice problems among teachers. Differences by gender and teacher characteristics. *Journal of Voice, 12,* (3), 328–334.

Stemple, J. C. (1996). Voice disorders: An introduction. *Language, Speech, and Hearing Services in Schools, 27,* 239.

St. Louis, K., & Myers, F. (1998). A synopsis of cluttering and its treatment. [On-line] Available: http://www.mankato.msus.edu/dept/ comdis/isad/papers/stlouis/html

Stuttering Foundation of America. (1999). *If you think your child stutters: A guide for parents.* Memphis, TN: Author.

Swan, A. (1993). Helping children who stutter: What teachers need to know. *Childhood Education, 69,* (3), 138–141.

Thomas, P., & Carmack, F. (1990). *Speech and language: Detecting and correcting special needs.* Boston: Allyn & Bacon.

Van Riper, C., (1982). *The nature of stuttering.* Englewood Cliffs. NJ: Prentice-Hall.

Vocal rehabilitation after total laryngectomy. (n.d.). (On-line). Available: http://www.origin8.nl/ medical/index.htm

Weiss, C., & Lillywhite, H. (1981). *Communicative disorders: Prevention & early intervention.* St. Louis: C. V. Mosby.

White, E. B. (1970). *The trumpet of the swan.* New York: Harper & Row.

Yairi, E. (1998). Is the basis for stuttering genetic? *American Speech Language and Hearing Association, 70,* (1), 29–32.

Yairi, E., Ambrose, N. G., Paden, E. P., & Throneburg, R. D. (1996). Predictive factors of persistence and recovering: Pathways of childhood stuttering. *Journal of Communication Disorders, 29,* 51–77.

9

Problems of Hearing: Identification and Remediation

Martha S. Lue

Chapter Objectives

On completion of this chapter, the reader will be able to:

- Describe the hearing mechanism, nature and severity of hearing problems, types and incidences of hearing problems; and
- Develop and implement strategies that the classroom teacher might employ in working with students who exhibit problems of hearing.

- At age three, Lisa was a normal, active little girl who showed a slight difficulty in speech. By three and a half, the speech difficulty became more pronounced. Lisa was taken for evaluation for early intervention due to apparent speech, language, and behavior difficulties when interacting with her peers. The evaluation revealed a hearing loss in her left ear. At this time, the loss was described as one for all audible sounds below 30 decibels. She began attending school in an early intervention program where she dropped further behind her peers and her problems began to escalate.

By five years of age she was placed in a self-contained classroom for students with emotional handicaps because of "non-compliant and combative behaviors." The school system that she attended did not do any further evaluations on the hearing loss. At six, she was taken to a hearing specialist who specialized in working with children. The results showed a hearing loss in both ears for sounds from 80dB and below. After the family moved from the area, she was reevaluated at a local hospital and was found to have a condition called **otospongiosis.**

Otospongiosis is a condition in which deposits of spongy bone exist between the stapes and the oval window in the ear. It occurs in about 1 in 1000 people. As the spongy bone tissue grows, the stapes becomes immobilized and can no longer transmit sensations to the inner ear. Before having surgery, Lisa attended a special program for children at Gallaudet University for a year to help with her speech and acquisition of language. The surgery that restored her hearing removed the spongy tissue in the right ear and also removed the stapes and replaced them with an artificial device in the left ear. The doctor who performed the surgery said, however, that there was a possibility that she will lose her hearing later in life due to regrowth of spongy tissue.

Now, at age twelve, she is on "monitor" in a regular education environment and attends speech therapy once a week. Lisa has exceeded what was expected of her. Her reading comprehension and written language are now on a ninth-grade level and her verbal expression is on a low seventh-grade level. She does have a hearing aid, which she does not use, for her right ear. She says she would rather hear muffled sounds than the noises through a hearing aid. Another one of her favorite excuses is that when she uses the aid she hears sounds from all over the classroom at once and that interrupts her thinking. As with most twelve-year-old females, she is concerned with how she looks and uses any excuse not to use the aid.

- Mara is a ten-year-old fifth-grade student with Wardensberg syndrome. Characteristics of this syndrome may include: profound deafness, lack of tear ducts, soft teeth and nails, and a streak of white through one's hair, shortened arms, underdeveloped hands, and above average intelligence. (An estimated 5 percent of individuals with congenital deafness have this genetic disease.) Mara is well-liked in the classroom, has many friends, and plays baseball on the Challengers Team for children with disabilities. She is able to learn and share her ideas. Though Mara can understand sign language and demonstrates excellent speech-reading skills, she becomes frustrated when attempting to express herself. With the assistance of the Augmentative School Specialist at the school district, the school-based team, along with Mara and her parents, will develop an individual education program (IEP) to include her in a "least restrictive environment" (LRE).

This child is a special case, her teacher reports. She is a fifth grader, which means that her appearance is becoming more important to her. She already felt different enough with her white and black hair, her underdeveloped hands, and with the cochlear implant device she wears. What could the instructional team find for this student with high intelligence to use for communication that was "cool"? She is deaf, so she would need to see what the machine was "saying." If the augmentative device involved typing, the keys had to be far apart and sensitive to her light touch. The groups finally decided on a Touch-Talker, a device that would allow Mara to type in a message to be voiced, great for interaction in the mainstream. She can type her lessons, print them, and hold conversations with nonsigning people.

- A college student with a hearing impairment has this story to tell.

> My hearing loss went undetected until the third grade because my grandmother is hearing impaired, which caused everyone in the family to speak loudly when they talked. Plus my mother taught me to read and write before I entered kindergarten.
>
> As I went through grade school, I encountered lots of problems with my teachers. I still remember my first week of kindergarten when my teacher made me sit in the back of the room in time out because I, as she told my principal, was not interested in learning because I never participated with other students. After that incident, my mother would accompany me to elementary school for the first week of each semester and pop up unexpectedly to make sure the teacher was not treating me like an outcast because I was different. But things were no better in middle school.
>
> During my middle-school years, my mother had to come to have a conference with my teachers frequently. My band teacher didn't want me to be in his class at all. He honestly told my mother that he "never had a hearing impaired child or handicapped child in music." My mother responded by saying, "And I never had a hearing-impaired child before. This is my firstborn and I love her too much to turn my back on her. I learned that she learns just as well as a normal child. She just needs her lessons amplified." To this day I thank my band teacher for his determination to teach me to play the clarinet and to love music. During my high school years, I was faced with social situations. All through kindergarten through sixth grade, I only talked to my grandmother and mother, and a very few relatives. I was always in my room, either doing homework or reading lots of books. I didn't have any friends outside the family until ninth grade, when I met my first true friend. We became fast friends and she came to

understand my impairment, and because we had every class together because of our last names, she even took extra notes to help me hear what was going on.

As a result of my background, I have learned to read everything I can, speak slowly and as clearly as possible, and not to be afraid of my speech or handicap. That is why I strive to be the best Exceptional Student teacher or Deaf teacher I can be so I can help children whom society calls "different or abnormal" to be the best they can be.

Reports show that more than 28 million people in the United States have some form of hearing loss (Goldberg, 1993). Approximately 4 percent of people under forty-five years of age and 29 percent of those sixty-five and older suffer a hearing loss. One out of every six elementary students might be expected to suffer from a hearing loss. The ASHA Committee on Infant Hearing (1998) estimates that 7 to 12 percent of all newborn babies are at risk for hearing impairment.

While the nature and severity of the hearing loss may vary, the loss of hearing is one of the most damaging losses that can occur in one's life. A significant hearing loss, as in the cases in the vignettes, has far-reaching effects on all aspects of an individual's development—cognitive, linguistic, and social/emotional.

Reflection

In 1994, a young woman with a profound sensorineural hearing loss was crowned Miss America. How do you think that this event has contributed to the general public's understanding of individuals who may require some form of hearing modification or adaptation in their daily lives?

This chapter will present an overview of hearing, the hearing process, and resulting problems in students when the auditory system fails to develop or is damaged. Topics to be discussed include: the hearing mechanism, nature and severity of hearing problems, types and incidence of hearing problems, and strategies for the classroom teacher in working with students who exhibit problems of hearing. An introduction to the area, the first section will contain an explanation of some basic terms and concepts helpful in understanding this chapter.

The Hearing Mechanism

The ear is, by far, one of the most complex and important organs. Knowledge of the function of the ear relative to sound will provide insight into the complex process of hearing. It is difficult to understand speech as a physiological process without considering the structure of the hearing mechanism, which enables one to receive speech and monitor his or her own speech production. By hearing the pragmatically appropriate speech in others and in various situations, children develop sound–symbol relationships and linguistic structures.

The Ear and Related Structures

The human ear is divided into three major sections: the outer (external) ear, the middle ear, and the inner ear. Although the outer ear is usually considered the least important for hearing and the inner ear the most important, each element is important to the speech and hearing process.

Outer Ear (External Ear).   The outer ear, the visible part of the ear, includes the pinna (auricle) and auditory meatus canal. The function of the outer ear is to assist in the funneling or "gathering in" of sound. The pinna funnels the sound to the ear canal and helps localize sounds. The auditory meatus canal acts as a resonator of the sound it receives and it also boosts the high-frequency sounds. The canal is lined with skin. The outer portion of the canal contains numerous glands, which produce cerumen (earwax). The outer canal is open and, hence, filled with air, and is primarily a place of acoustical energy. At the end of the canal is the tympanic membrane (eardrum). The tympanic membrane, a thin, elastic cone-shaped organ, separates the outer and middle ear.

Middle Ear.   The middle ear contains three moving bones, the ossicles: hammer (malleus), anvil (incus), and stirrups (stapes). The malleus, the largest of the ossicles, is directly attached to the eardrum. The incus, called the "intermediate communicating link" (Seikel, King, & Drumright, 1997), serves as a bridge between the malleus and the stapes. The other end of the stapes is inserted into the oval window, a small opening that leads to the inner ear. The movement of the ossicles transmits vibrations of the eardrum from the middle ear to the inner ear. It amplifies sound about 30 dB. The energy that causes the vibrations of the eardrum begins, of course, with the airflow in the outer ear.

Eustachian Tube.   The eustachian tube connects the middle ear with the nasopharynx. The nasopharynx is a part of the back of the throat; it opens into the nasal passage. The eustachian tube helps to maintain air pressure at an effective level in the middle ear where the tympanum is exposed to external pressure from the air moving into the ear. The tube is often a source of infections in the middle ear because of its connections to the throat. Excessive buildup of pressure within the middle ear may cause the eardrum to rupture.

Inner Ear.   Often called the *labyrinth* because of its resemblance to a maze of passageways, the inner ear begins with the oval window, a small opening in the bone that houses the inner ear. Other parts of the inner ear include the semicircular canals, the cochlea, the organ of Corti, and the vestibule. The vestibule contains the three semicircular canals and is responsible for balance, sense of body position, and movement. The cochlea, a snail-shaped organ, is concerned with hearing. The organ of Corti, sometimes called the *essential* or *end organ* of hearing, contains several thousand hair cells, specialized cells that respond to sound. The inner ear is filled with fluids, endolymph and perilymph. The parts of the ear are illustrated in Figure 9.1.

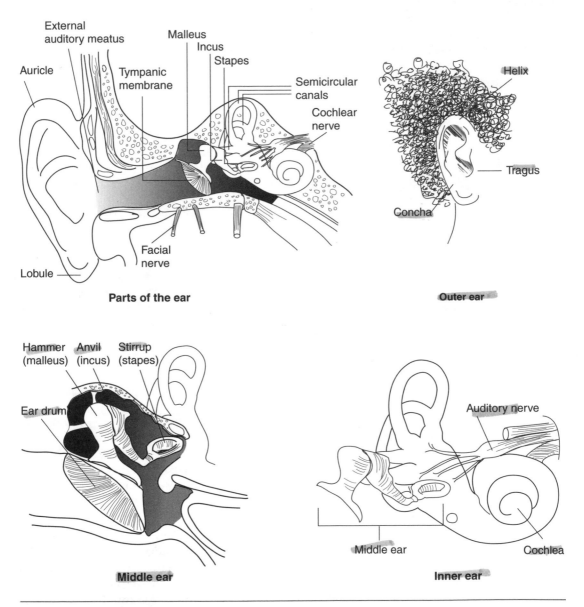

FIGURE 9.1 *Parts of the Ear*

Courtesy of John Albritton, M. D.

Eighth Cranial Nerve and the Brain.   Known as the auditory or acoustic nerve, the eighth cranial nerve connects the inner ear and the brain. The eighth cranial nerve, therefore, transmits the sounds that the brain interprets.

Description of the Hearing Process

The sense of hearing is one of our most complex sensory processes. "Hearing," notes Skinner (1985), "is a basic process from which human communication evolves" (p. 171). Without this functioning biological system, sound would not be heard and understood, thus communication would be greatly impaired. As you review the complexity of the hearing process, you will quickly realize that it is a sense that should never be taken for granted. The following represents a brief description of the hearing process.

- Sound energy, originating as vibration and transmitted through the air, is captured by the outer ear, which funnels the sound inside through the auditory meatus canal.
- There the sound energy strikes the **tympanic membrane** (eardrum), causing it to vibrate.
- These vibrations are transmitted across the middle ear space to the inner ear by three small bones (or ossicles), known as the **malleus, incus,** and **stapes.**
- In addition to serving as a conductor for sound energy, the tympanic membrane and middle ear ossicles amplify the sound. The stapes transmit the amplified vibrations through the oval window.
- The vibration transmitted by the stapes induces motion in the fluids of the cochlea that fill the inner ear.
- The vibratory fluid motion, with associated hair cells, ultimately causes a nerve impulse, which is transmitted to the brain via cranial nerve VIII (auditory nerve). Here the sounds can be interpreted as meaningful information.

In summary, sound energy is funneled into the outer ear through the auditory meatus canal into the middle ear. Through the oval window, these waves are carried into the fluids of the inner ear. These fluids move the hair cells, which in turn allow the brain to differentiate between these sounds.

Dimensions of Hearing

Sounds are measured along two dimensions: loudness and pitch. The presence of hearing loss is determined by observing an individual's response to sound. That is done informally in social settings and formally in clinical testing. In a laboratory, the assessment is made with measured sounds in a controlled environment. The frequency of the sound (high versus low pitch) is measured in **hertz** (Hz). Hertz are usually measured from 125 Hz ("low" sounds) to 8,000 Hz ("high" sounds). Studies report that 80 percent of all speech sounds fall between 500 and

2,000 Hz. Normal young human beings can hear sounds between 20 and 20,000 Hz, but other mammals—bats, dolphins, and whales, for example—can hear frequencies of a much higher level.

Activity

With the use of an encyclopedia or a specialized textbook on hearing, determine the frequency range for several different animals.

Intensity of sound (loud vs. quiet) is measured in **decibels** (dB) (named for Alexander Graham Bell). Audiologists, professionals in the science dealing with hearing impairments, their detection, and remediation, are usually concerned with measuring the sensitivity to sounds from 0 to about 110 dB. It is believed, specifically, that the ability to hear across the frequency between 0 and 40 dB is critical for the development of normal speech and language. Table 9.1 indicates the decibel levels of several sounds commonly heard in the environment.

The lowest intensity of a sound needed to stimulate the auditory system is called the hearing threshold level **(HTL).** Speech sounds in normal conversation with the speakers five feet apart fall between 20 and 50 dB. Factors that affect the ability to hear certain sounds are: distance from the source, background noises, and acoustics of the room. Intensity, note Eisenson and Ogilvie (1983), varies directly as the amount of energy applied to the body capable of vibration. An individual's *threshold for hearing* is the level at which he or she can first detect a sound, i.e., how intense a sound must be before the person can detect it.

TABLE 9.1   *Decibel Levels of Several Environmental Sounds*

Source	*Perception/Hearing*	*Sound Level (dB)*
Whisper	Just audible	10
Rustle of leaves		30
Normal conversation	Comfortable	50
Auto traffic		60
Window air-conditioner	Loud	80
Snowmobile/Motorcycle		95
Power lawn mower	Very loud	100
Pneumatic jackhammer/Chain saw		110
Rock music		115
Oxygen torch	Uncomfortably loud	120

Northern, J., & Lemme, M. (1986). Hearing and auditory disorders. In G. Shames & E. Wiig (Eds.), *Human communication disorders* (p. 418). Columbus, OH: Merrill. Reprinted with permission.

Nature/Types of Hearing Loss

Hearing Impairments Defined

People with hearing problems are generally divided into two groups according to the severity of their hearing loss: **deaf** and **hearing impaired.** The term *deaf* is commonly used to describe those individuals who exhibit a hearing loss of 90 dB or greater. Specifically, the Individuals with Disabilities Education Act (IDEA) defines deaf as:

> A hearing impairment which is so severe that the child is impaired in processing linguistic information through hearing, with or without amplification, which adversely affects educational performance.

For the deaf individual, even with the use of a hearing aid, the hearing loss is too great for the understanding of speech.

While *hearing impaired* is often used to cover all hearing losses, the term is used specifically to describe a hearing loss less than that of deaf persons. Individuals described as hearing impaired have residual hearing sufficient for successful processing of linguistic information through audition. Special adaptations or technological aids, such as the use of a hearing aid, may be needed (Brill, MacNeil, & Newman, 1986). In reference to the terms describing hearing impairments, it has been reported that the terms *deaf* and *hard of hearing* are preferred in the deaf community in the United States, rather than the term *hearing impaired* (Harris, Van Zandt, & Rees, 1997).

Causes

Hearing losses are also typed according to the source of the loss. They are usually classified as three general types: **conductive** (those involving the outer and middle ear), **sensorineural** (usually involving the inner ear), and mixed (involving both conductive and sensorineural loss). A fourth classification, central auditory nerve loss, often does not show up on routine hearing tests. A fifth, nonorganic impairment, is receiving more attention in the research literature. Each will be described briefly.

Conductive Loss.   This type of hearing loss, usually mild, occurs when there is interference of any sort in the transmission of sound from the external auditory meatus canal to the middle ear. Any material that blocks the passageway can cause a conductive hearing loss (Martin, 1997). A conductive hearing loss is generally reversible and can be treated medically or surgically. Causes of a conductive hearing loss can include:

- **Tinnitus,** a constant, or almost constant, ringing or whistling in the ear;
- Foreign objects or debris that block the external auditory meatus canal;

- **Otitis media,** the largest single cause of hearing loss, a middle-ear infection, fluid in the middle ear, often associated with upper respiratory infections;
- Cerumen (ear wax) impaction;
- Congenital abnormalities of the ear, including atresia (a condition in which the external canal may be completely closed);
- **Otosclerosis,** a disease in which the stapes become fixated or rigid in the oval window. This condition appears to be more common in women than in men (Hedge, 1995).

Conductive hearing losses appear to be common in children with a variety of disabilities (Howard, Williams, Port, & Lepper, 1997; Hilt, 1998). Included are children with Down, Treacher-Collins, Ushers, Pierre Robin, and Cri-du-Chat syndromes and children with cleft lips and palates.

Sensorineural Hearing Loss.   This type of hearing loss occurs when there is damage to the hair cells of the cochlea or the auditory nerve fibers, which prevents the brain from receiving the neural impulses of sound. It is generally irreversible; hearing usually cannot be restored through medical or surgical treatment. Causes may include:

- viral or bacterial infections (e.g., meningitis, syphilis);
- drug toxicity (taken by the pregnant mother or the child);
- excessive noise exposure (prolonged exposure to intense noise such as loud music, firecrackers, or explosives);
- **presbycusis,** a hearing loss incurred due to the effect of aging; and
- head trauma

Neonates and premature infants may be at risk of acquiring sensorineural hearing losses. Causes may include asphyxia of infants during delivery, which can damage the cochlea, high bilirubin levels, which may result in severe jaundice, cerebral hemorrhage, and apnea. Cytomegalovirus (CMV), the leading congenital nonhereditary cause of sensorineural hearing loss in children, affects an average of 1 percent of all live births within the United States (McCollister, Simpson, Dahle, Pass, Fowler, Amos, & Boll, 1996). Cytomegalovirus is a group of highly specific viruses characterized by jaundice, microcephaly, mental retardation, and hearing loss. It is detectable in utero through amniocentesis but is said to be difficult to diagnose (Hardman, Drew, & Egan, 1999).

Mixed Hearing Loss.   This type of hearing loss results when both the middle and inner ear are not functioning properly. The problem occurs simultaneously from both the conductive and sensorineural mechanisms. The cause of the mixed hearing loss, however, may stem from two completely different sources. The conductive portion of the hearing loss may be reversible.

Central Auditory Nerve Loss.   This type of loss occurs when there is faulty interpretation of sound information sent to the brain. In individuals with central auditory nerve loss, the individual may hear, that is, the ear itself works properly, but cannot understand speech under such difficult listening conditions as background noises. Causes may include sharp, severe blows to the head, tumors, brain damage, or degenerative diseases affecting the central auditory structure.

Nonorganic Hearing Loss.   A nonorganic hearing loss is one that has no obvious physical or structural cause. Severe emotional traumas, such as having psychological shocks and witnessing violent acts, can all lead to nonorganic hearing losses.

Reflection

What are some environmental noise sources that may be damaging to the ear? Reflect on how you can protect your ears from being damaged in such situations.

Language Development and Hearing Loss

It is believed that the period of development from birth to approximately three years of age is a critical period for the development of normal speech and language. Thus, the domain most directly affected by hearing loss in infancy is language. Quigley and Kretschmer (1982) have identified several factors that influence the development of language in the presence of a hearing loss: degree of hearing loss, age of onset of loss, slope of hearing loss, age of identification of hearing loss, age of habilitation, amount of habilitation, and type of habilitation.

Unilateral versus Bilateral Hearing Loss

For some children, the hearing loss occurs on one side, that is, in one ear. This loss is referred to as *unilateral.* For other children, the hearing loss occurs on both sides or in both ears. This loss is called *bilateral hearing loss.* It is evident that a unilateral loss has less serious impact than a bilateral loss. In most cases, children with unilateral hearing loss typically develop language normally and perform at their age level on communication tasks.

Children who exhibit a hearing loss and are identified early and receive early intervention show greater receptive and expressive language gains than those who receive no or later intervention. Two terms are generally used to describe the periods at which a hearing loss begins—prelingual or postlingual. A **prelingual hearing loss** develops before the onset of speech and language. It is during this period that language is most affected. A **postlingual hearing loss** develops after speech and language have been acquired. Martin and Noble (1994) have reported several screening methods that can be used to detect a hearing loss in children, including the Crib-O-Gram, the neonatal auditory response cradle, and the *ABC* test.

Two other terms that you will need to be familiar with are: **congenitally deaf** and **adventitiously deaf.** Congenitally deaf is a condition in which hearing loss exists at or before birth. Adventitiously deaf is a hearing loss that occurs after birth and is due to injury or disease.

Reflection

Do you think it is important for the classroom teacher to know the cause, type, and severity of hearing loss that the child might exhibit? Justify your answer.

Educational Approaches

Helping a hearing impaired child communicate on a day-to-day basis requires a lot of thought. No one approach will work for all children. Two prominent issues guiding your decision are those regarding habilitation and rehabilitation. Both of these topics will be readdressed under the discussion of educational implications.

Habilitation versus Rehabilitation

For some children, hearing loss occurs from the time of birth or before normal language development. These youngsters require a management program called *habilitation*. For those who acquire a hearing loss after language and speech have been established, the prescribed management program is called *rehabilitation*.

As a classroom teacher, you will be concerned about the mode of communication in the classroom that will best serve the child with a hearing impairment's education and general social adjustment (Stuckless & Birch, 1997). Several augmentative communication systems may be prescribed for a child with the day-to-day supervision task assigned to his or her teacher. Some of the common educational approaches designed to assist a child to communicate are: auditory–oral, manual, and total communication. Each will be discussed briefly.

Auditory–Oral.   Use of speech and hearing to communicate. Children are taught to communicate through speech and to make use of their residual (available) hearing or augment it with hearing aids and other assistive devices.

Manual Communication.   Use of hand movements to represent words. It includes any of a number of sign language systems, including American Sign Language (ASL), Signing Exact English (SEE), and finger spelling. An example of the American manual alphabet is illustrated in Figure 9.2.

The manual alphabet as the receiver sees it:

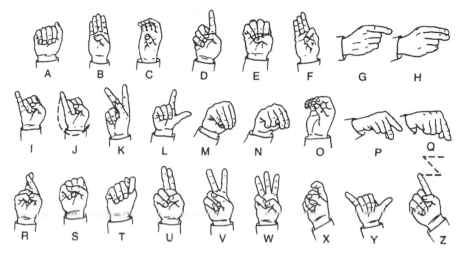

The manual alphabet as the sender sees it:

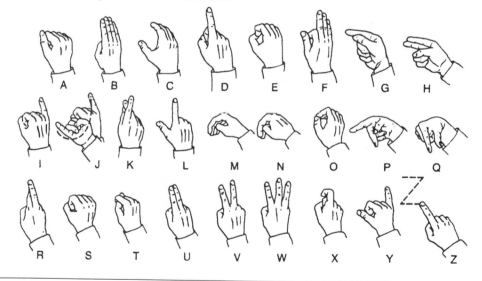

FIGURE 9.2 *The American Manual Alphabet*

From M. L. Hardman, C. J. Drew, & M. W. Egan (1999). In *Human exceptionality. Society, school, and family* (6th ed., p. 414). Boston: Allyn & Bacon. Reprinted with permission.

Total Communication. This involves use of a combination of both auditory–oral and manual systems. In addition, with this approach, the interpretation of facial expressions, body language, and gestures is taught and speech reading and writing may be used to communicate.

> *Activity*
>
> Visit a class, a clinic, a school, or other setting where signing is used or ask someone who signs to visit your class for a demonstration.

Educational Implications for Youngsters with Hearing Impairments

Habilitation

In those children requiring habilitation, consideration should be given to the onset, type, and extent of the hearing loss in young children. It is important to note that habilitative efforts are quite individualized, and may depend primarily on the extent of the hearing loss and the age of the child. In all cases, the classroom teacher should work very closely with the trained speech, language, or audiological professional, as well as the parents, to ensure that the child's educational needs are met.

> *Activity*
>
> Several hearing aids are advertised on TV, in magazines, in newspapers, and in professional journals. Locate at least two advertisements on which to comment. Identify the specific feature the aid is promoting—amplification, clarity, ease of use, cosmetic. Describe strengths and weaknesses that you perceive in the ad.

Mild Hearing Loss (15–40 dB).   For children with mild hearing losses, vowel sounds are heard clearly, but voiceless consonants (e.g., /p/, /k/, /t/, /s/, /f/) may be missed. The child in the classroom with such a loss should be given preferential seating. Other accommodations to be made include teaching the child to develop basic listening competencies, to learn to listen critically, and to watch others closely as part of an auditory training program (Boone & Plante, 1993). Northern and Downs (1989) add that a child with a hearing loss of 25 dB–40 dB should always be fitted with a hearing aid.

Several types of hearing aids are available, including the body type (microphone and amplifier unit are worn somewhere on the front of the body); behind the ear (the aid is hooked behind the ear with sound being fed by a short piece of plastic tubing to an ear mold fitting the ear opening); in the ear (the aid is inserted in the ear just as an ear mold would be); and in the ear canal (entire aid may be worn in the ear canal).

Moderate Hearing Loss (40–65 dB).   The student misses almost all of the speech sounds at conversational level, but can learn language with the help of a hearing aid. Short, unstressed words, such as prepositions, as well as word endings, /-s/ and /-ed/, may be particularly difficult to hear. The child must be taught speech reading skills and learn to communicate by watching others closely and using facial expression and gesture for interpretation and added understanding.

Severe Hearing Loss (65–90 dB).   For the severely hearing impaired student, language and speech will not develop spontaneously, but with early special education and amplification and with hearing aids these children may eventually function as well as hard-of-hearing persons. For speech and voice training for the hearing-impaired child, working with trained speech–language professionals is a must.

Profound Hearing Loss (90+ dB).   For the profoundly hearing-impaired child, language and speech must be learned by intensive special education. With amplification, profoundly hearing-impaired children may be able to hear the rhythmic patterns of speech, their own vocalizations, and loud environmental sounds. A child diagnosed with anacusis, a loss that exceeds 110 dB, has a total hearing loss. Powerful hearing aids can often be fitted that make use of any residual hearing that the child might have. In a few cases, a new treatment, the cochlear implant, is being used. In this surgical procedure, electrodes are implanted into the cochlea of the inner ear. An internal receiver, a microphone, is implanted in bone behind the outer ear. Through a complicated process, eventually external auditory impulses are carried as neural impulses by the auditory nerve to the hearing center at the base of the brain (Boone & Plante, 1993). The vast majority of candidates for this surgery are congenitally deaf; over 90 percent of them have normally hearing parents who want their children to hear and speak (O'Donoghue, 1999). After implants are placed, extensive audio/vocal training is necessary to accomplish this goal.

Reflection

The National Association for the Deaf states that "deaf people don't need to be fixed," and disavows the use of a cochlear implant. As a parent of a profoundly hearing-impaired child, present your reactions to this response.

Rehabilitation Programs

For children who have developed normal speech and language before the onset of the hearing loss, a program of rehabilitation should be established. Rehabilitation issues that need to be considered include: the fitting of a hearing aid, an aural rehabilitation program, and any need for psychological counseling (Boone & Plante, 1993). The classroom teacher, with the assistance of the trained speech, language, or audiological professional, should work collaboratively with all related disciplines to ensure that the child's educational needs are being met.

Early Identification and Behavioral Indications of a Possible Hearing Loss

On average, children who are deaf are identified at approximately fifteen months of age. Children who are hard of hearing, however, are not usually identified until over a year later (Meadow-Orlans, Sass-Lehrer, Scott-Olsen, & Mertens, 1998). It is critical that early identification of both categories take place for a number of reasons, including recognition and development of age appropriate language and communication skills, as well as the development of appropriate social skills.

While it is believed that nearly all children with severe hearing losses are identified before they reach school, this may certainly not be the case for a child who might exhibit a mild hearing impairment. Therefore, children might enter school without having had a hearing impairment detected, or they may have a loss after they enter school. As a classroom teacher, you may be one of the first to suspect that a child might be experiencing difficulty in hearing. Here are some behaviors to watch for:

- Failing to respond to a statement or request, even when called by name or when the child appears to be paying attention;
- Consistently asking for classroom directions, games rules, or portions of conversations to be repeated;
- Seldom initiating conversation, not volunteering in the class, and not wanting to share during show and tell;
- Answering very simple questions incorrectly or performing one task after being told to do another;
- Child's complaining of tinnitus (whistling or ringing in ears);
- Noticeable discharge from ear;
- Constant complaints of dizziness;
- Turning TV too loud for others;
- A history of hearing loss in family;
- Consistently tugging on ears;
- Frequent absences from school due to earaches, sinus congestion, allergies, and related conditions;
- Frequent imitation of other students' behaviors in the classroom;
- Spending most of the time daydreaming or engaging in solitary play;
- Showing aggression toward other people or objects;
- Child turning his or her ear to the sound source;
- Child intently watching the face or mouth of the speaker in order to speech-read;
- Speech and/or language development delayed or very difficult to understand.

If a child exhibits any of these symptoms more than occasionally, an evaluation of hearing should be recommended. Keep in mind, however, that some of these behaviors may be indicative of other kinds of problems. This list represents indicators that might warrant further investigation, rather than conclusive proof that a hearing loss exists.

Assessing Individuals with a Hearing Loss

Charles Van Riper (1994), a pioneer in the field of speech-language pathology, recounts the tremendous strides the field of audiology has made.

> When I started the first speech clinic in 1936, there were no audiometers back then, so when I suspected a hearing loss, I measured it by calibrating the office by painting white lines across it, which would represent how far away from the tuning forks a normally hearing person could no longer hear the sound . . . There was another line, one in red paint, that represented the distance from an alarm clock where a normal hearing person could no longer hear it tick. (p. 37)

Now with increased sophistication in electronic devices, testing can be done more accurately and definitively.

Hearing Assessment in Students

Hearing is formally tested by a procedure called *pure tone audiometry.* Professionally trained persons, such as an audiologist or a speech-language pathologist in most cases, will conduct the formal testing. The tester uses an **audiometer,** an electronic device that generates sounds at different levels of intensity and frequency. Simple instructions are given to the child before testing—raise your hand when you hear the sound, lower it when you don't.

As members of an instructional team, a teacher should be able to get professional assistance for any specific questions from a speech-language pathologist and an audiologist.

- To begin with, hearing is tested using earphones or loud speakers that send sounds to the ear.
- Each ear is tested separately. This is important because a hearing loss can occur in one or both ears. The tester will present a variety of pure tones, ranging from 0 to about 110 dB and 125 to 8,000 Hz, until the level of intensity (in dB) is reached when the individual can detect the tone at a number of frequencies.
- The audiometer can produce tones ranging from a very low frequency level of 125 Hz through 250, 500, 1000, 2000, 3000, 4000, 6000, and 8000 Hz.
- The tester gradually increases the intensity until the child signals hearing.
- For each of these levels of frequency, there is an assessment of the degree of hearing loss. This is placed on an **audiogram,** a graph of hearing sensitivity.

As was previously stated, the amount of hearing loss is determined by measuring the hearing threshold. The shape or pattern of the hearing level threshold is called the configuration. "X's" are used to represent the left ear and "O's" are used to represent the right ear's configuration.

- If testing reveals a hearing loss, another device, called a *bone vibrator* (bone conduction), is used to determine the type of hearing loss.
- If additional testing is needed, the child is referred to one or more of the members of the hearing professional team.

Members of the Hearing Profession Team

There may be several members on the hearing profession team. Each plays a distinct, yet collaborative, role as they provide services for children. It is important that you are familiar with the duties of each of these trained professionals because they can serve as a ready resource to assist you in working with the child with a hearing impairment. As Van Riper and Erickson (1996) noted, "the most effective rehabilitation of individuals with hearing loss takes place when skilled and knowledgeable specialists work cooperatively together and with the individual and his or her family" (p. 451). Physicians who specialize in treating ear and hearing problems are called **otologists** or **otolaryngologists.** An otologist is a specialist in ear diseases. An otolarnygologist is one who studies the ear, the upper respiratory tract, and the treatment of their diseases (Dox, Melloni, & Eisner, 1985). These individuals can ascertain whether the hearing loss can be improved with medical or surgical treatment. **Audiologists** are educational professionals who specialize in evaluating the level of hearing loss and conducting hearing tests. They may also recommend the use of hearing aids or assistive listening devices, if appropriate.

Audiologists hold a master's or doctoral degree in audiology. They also hold a Certificate of Clinical Competence from the American Speech-Language-Hearing Association.

Americans with Disabilities Act (ADA) and Individuals with Hearing Impairments

The Americans with Disabilities Act (ADA, Public Law 101-336), signed into law on July 26, 1990, and reauthorized in 1997, is considered one of the most important pieces of civil rights legislation for individuals with disabilities. Among its components are provisions for opportunities for consultations and provision of assistive devices. The Americans with Disabilities Act (ADA) requires that all school-sponsored activities (sports, plays, concerts) be accessible to all students.

Technology is being used increasingly as a way to reduce or remove communications barriers through assistive aids. Jensema (1994) has delineated several technological advances that seem to positively impact the lives of hearing impaired persons. Among those described are relay services, bulletin board/online services, electronic mail, video telephones, and speech recognition.

Use of Interpreters in the Educational Setting

The most common resource provided to youngsters who are deaf or hard of hearing in an inclusive classroom setting is the provision of interpreter services (Luetke-Stahlman, 1998). As we move toward a more inclusive educational environment, students of varying levels of hearing abilities, from the child with a moderate loss to the child with a profound hearing loss, may be educated in a general or special education setting. A small number of these students may require the assistance of an interpreter. Interpreters are highly trained professionals who may accompany some students with hearing impairments to assist them in communicating. The interpreter conveys all oral communication to the deaf student and voices all signed responses the student may make, thus enabling the student to participate actively during class sessions. Other duties may include tutoring, assisting regular and special education teachers, keeping records, and supervising students with hearing impairments (Heward, 2000). Some general information about interpreters is found in Table 9.2.

TABLE 9.2 *Interpreters in Education Settings*

General Guidelines	• Include the interpreter as a member of the IEP team in terms of the communication needs of the students.
	• Request an interpreter (i.e., do not let parents interpret for their children) for certain important situations (e.g., transition planning meetings).
	• Supervise the interpreter if this person is involved with additional classroom tasks.
	• Meet with the assigned interpreter regularly to discuss the needs of the student and review ongoing communication patterns.
	• Evaluate the effectiveness of interpreters.
Specific Suggestions	• Allow the interpreter to be positioned so that the student can easily see both the teacher (or media) and the interpreter.
	• Prepare the interpreter for the topic(s) that will be covered and the class format that will be followed.
	• Provide copies of all visual materials (e.g., overhead transparencies) before class begins.
	• Be sensitive to the "time-lag" factor associated with interpreting—the few-word delay that the interpreter lags behind the spoken message, used to ensure the student's understanding of the communication.
	• Program breaks in lecturing if at all possible.
	• Limit the teacher's movement so that the student can see the interpreter and teacher without difficulty.
	• Check student understanding regularly—ensure that the student does not fake understanding.

From T. E. C. Smith, E. A. Polloway, J. R. Patton, & C. A. Dowdy. (1995). In *Teaching students with special needs in inclusive settings* (p. 198). Boston: Allyn & Bacon. Reprinted with permission.

Parents of Children with Hearing Impairments

It has been reported that parents of over three-fourths of children who are deaf have no previous experience with deafness. Subsequently, these parents are for the most part unaware of the challenges they will face in both communicating and educating the child (Moestick, 1998). They also may be unaware of the services available to them and their child(ren).

Technology and the Child with a Hearing Impairment

Technology provides the hearing impaired with services such as speech recognition systems, which have the capacity to provide input, and TDD relay services, which eliminate operator assistance and provide speaker-independent, portable, and continuous speech language recognition. These systems function as natural language processors, going far beyond simple speech recognition. AT&T, in 1994, introduced a system that provides speech recognition operator assistance to the general public (Davila, 1994).

In 1992, IBM introduced the Phone Communicator, which connects the phone line to the personal computer. This product causes the computer screen to blink when a call comes in. When the person with a hearing impairment answers the phone, he or she types in a message, the computer translates it into speech for the caller, and the caller can respond by typing a return message on the telephone keypad. The computer software has word prediction and thus can guess what letters are actually being chosen (one of three) from the telephone's key pad with fairly good accuracy (Filipczak, 1993). This "prerecognition" speeds up the communication process. Speeding up written speech is always a goal for improved technology as the writing and reading of language is far slower than that of natural hearing.

The use of an FM listening system with a remote microphone has proven helpful for some students with hearing impairments. In this process, the student wears a hearing aid, while the teacher wears a microphone. Brackett (1997) notes that "by having the primary sound source close to the remote microphone, the signal is enhanced relative to the background noise to levels approximating those for optimal perception" (p. 356). Nussbaum (1988) found that in most classrooms that have students with hearing impairments, the use of the radio FM auditory trainer is employed. Mullis and Otwell (1998) remind us that the microphone is sensitive and teachers should not wear jewelry and certain articles of clothing that might cause the transmission of extraneous noises. Finally, the microphone should be turned off when it is not needed.

Reflection

What do you think that technology will hold for the person with a hearing impairment in the year 2030?

The Hard-of-Hearing Child in the Classroom

Strategies for Success

A hearing impairment, notes Luckner (1991), may "impose an invisible acoustic filter that impacts students' verbal language development and their reading and writing skills" (p. 302). Students with hearing problems may require modifications to the physical, social, and instructional environment in order for them to realize their fullest potential. Placement of students in various service delivery models depends on each student's language and communication ability, the severity of the hearing loss, educational abilities, and the presence of other disabilities (Mullis & Otwell, 1998). The following list, while far from being complete, represents a start as you anticipate modifying the environment for optimal gains. Seek the assistance of specialists in the field (speech-language pathologists, audiologists) who can provide further guidance. Keep in mind that each student is unique. Capitalize on the strengths that each child, whether hearing impaired or not, brings to the classroom (Eisenson & Ogilvie, 1983).

Activities
- **Many videos and books are available to illustrate life experiences of persons with hearing impairments. Begin to develop your own list.**
- **Invite a parent of a child with a hearing impairment to class.**

Working with Students with Hearing Losses

- Ensure that the child is seated where speakers are best seen and heard and where there is the least amount of interference (e.g., background noise). Make certain that this special seating does not further isolate or negatively single out the student.
- Ensure that no glare exists for the child as he or she watches a speaker or screen.
- When addressing the child with hearing impairments, speak naturally but somewhat more loudly and slowly than otherwise might be necessary.
- Use gestures freely but without exaggeration.
- Use visual materials and the blackboard for writing words, phrases, and sentences associated with the essential material of any oral presentation.
- Observe the child for signs of comprehension or confusion. If material is repeated, it should be an exact repetition.
- If the child is using a hearing aid, make certain that it works.

- Use Skinner and Shelton's (1985) SPEECH to teach parents and teachers how to communicate with hearing-impaired children.

  S = State the topic to be discussed;

  P = Pace your conversation at a moderate rate with occasional pauses to permit comprehension or for the child to catch up;

  E = Enunciate clearly, without exaggerated lip movement;

  E = Enthusiastically communicate, using body language and natural gestures;

  CH = Check comprehension before changing topics.

- Provide the child with as many similar auditory stimuli as you provide for those children without hearing impairments and encourage speech use as much as possible as a form of communication (Ling, 1990).

- Build on the child's existing communication skills.

- Social interaction with peers is important. Through the use of structured games, facilitate the hearing-impaired student's interaction with peers.

- When setting up learning centers in the classroom, post pictures of the rules of the learning center and place items that provide both visual and tactile stimulation in the center (Hoyett, 1994).

- Remove obstacles, such as chewing gum and food, when speaking.

- Realize that beards and mustaches can interfere with the student's ability to speech-read.

- Face the listener. Don't turn away when speaking.

- Get the listener's attention first by gently touching his or her shoulder, raising your finger, or giving some other type of beginning signal.

- Ask the listener who is hearing impaired what types of things would make the message easier to understand.

- To facilitate student involvement, use cooperative learning environments and a buddy system.

- Include a section of the lesson plan for listing several provisions for students with hearing impairment.

- Frequent comprehension monitoring is suggested. Ask comprehension questions. Students that are hearing impaired may not be aware of their comprehension difficulties; they may lack strategies necessary to request clarification.

- Hold students with hearing impairments to the same standards as their hearing peers, unless otherwise indicated.

- Use guest speakers who are hearing impaired. Students need to know that an impairment need not be viewed as a "disability."

- Teach hearing peers how to help the students who have hearing impairments.

Summary

The student with a hearing impairment may be at a distinct disadvantage in the acquisition of language. As an educator, you will need to be concerned about the extent to which the hearing loss affects the child's ability to speak and to understand spoken and written language. As we move toward a more inclusive educational environment, children with impairments of hearing ranging from mild to severe may be in your classroom. It then becomes your responsibility to learn as much about this topic as you can, recognizing the needs of individuals with hearing handicaps, and understanding the role that you play on this instructional team. Remember, you have professional colleagues to support you. While the topics discussed in this chapter have certainly not been exhaustive, the information will get you started to learn even more about this topic to find ways to help all students to learn.

References and Suggested Readings

Adams, J. W. (1988). *You and your hearing impaired child: A self instructional guide for parents.* Washington, DC: Clerc Books.

American Speech-Language-Hearing Association (ASHA). (1998). How do I know if I have a hearing loss. *Healthtouch online for better health* [online]. Available: http://www.healthtouch.com

American Speech-Language-Hearing Association (ASHA). (1998). Communication with people with hearing impairment. *Healthtouch online for better health* [online]. Available: http://www.healthtouch.com

Arnos, K. (1994). Heredity hearing loss. *New England Journal of Medicine, 331*(7), 469–470.

ASHA. (1993). Let's Talk. Hearing loss in children. *ASHA Journal,* vol 47–48.

ASHA Committee on Infant Hearing. (1998). Guidelines for the identification of hearing impairments in at risk infants age birth to six months. *ASHA, 30,* 61–64.

Atkins, D. (1987). Families and their hearing impaired children. *Volta Review, 89,* (5), 1–150.

Bess, F. A., & McConnell, F. E. (1981). *Audiology, education, and the hearing impaired child.* St. Louis: C. V. Mosby.

Boone, D. R., & Plante, E. (1993). *Human communication and its disorders* (2nd ed.). Englewood Cliffs, NJ: Prentice-Hall.

Brackett, D. (1997). Intervention for children with hearing impairments in general education settings. *Language, Speech, and Hearing Services in Schools, 28,* 355–361.

Brill, R. G., MacNeil, B., & Newman, L. R. (1986). Framework for appropriate programs for deaf children. *American Annals of the Deaf, 136,* (4), 339–343.

Chasin, M. (1998). Musicians and the prevention of hearing loss. *Hearing Journal, 51,* 10–16.

Conflitt, C. (1998). Early cognitive development and other sign language. *Exceptional Parent,* Vol. 40–41.

Crawford, M., & Studebader, G. (1998). Cytomegalovirus: A disease of hearing. *Hearing Journal, 43*(1), 25–30.

Davila, R. R. (1994) Technology and full participation for children and adults who are deaf. *American Annals of the Deaf, 139,* 6–9.

Demorest, M., and Erdman, S. (1936). Development of the communication profile for the hearing impaired. *Journal of Speech and Hearing Disorders, 52,* 129–143.

Dox, I., Melloni, B., & Eisner, G. (1985). *Melloni's illustrated medical dictionary* (2nd ed.). Baltimore: Williams & Wilkins.

Eisenson, J., & Ogilvie, M. (1983). *Communicative disorders in children* (5th ed.). New York: Macmillan.

Eiten, L. (1998). Fundamentals of Hearing. National Institute on Deafness and other Communication Disorders (NIDCD) Heredity Hearing Impairment Resource Registry. *Healthtouch* [online]. Available: http://www.healthtouch.com. Medical Strategies.

Filipczak, B. (1993). Adaptive technology for the disabled. *Training, 30*(3), 23–29.

Geers, A. E., Kozak, B., and Nicholas, J. G. (1994). Development of communicative function in your impaired and normally hearing children. *Volta Review, 96,* 113–135.

Goldberg, B. (1993). Universal hearing screening of newborns: An idea whose time has come. *ASHA, 35,* 63–64.

Gray, H. (1977). *Anatomy, descriptive & surgical* (15th ed.), T. P. Pick & R. Houden (Eds.). New York: Grameray.

Hardman, M., Drew, C., & Egan, M. (1999). *Human Exceptionality* (6th ed.). Boston: Allyn & Bacon.

Harris, L. K., Van Zandt, C. E., & Rees, T. (1997). Counseling needs of students who are deaf and hard of hearing. *The School Counselor, 44,* 271–279.

Hedge, M. (1995). *Introduction to communication disorders* (2nd ed.). Austin, TX: PRO-ED.

Heward, W. (2000). *Exceptional Children* (6th ed.). Englewood Cliffs, NJ: Merrill.

Hilt, G. (1998). Testing for hearing loss in children. *Exceptional Parent, 28*(5), 36–40.

Howard, M., & Hulit, L. (1992). Response patterns to central auditory tests and the clinical evaluation of language fundamentals, Revised: A pilot study. *Perceptual and Motor Skills, 74*(1), 120–123.

Howard, V., Williams, B., Port, P., & Lepper, C. (1997). *Very young children with special needs.* Upper Saddle River, NJ: Macmillan.

Hoyett, B. (1994). Involving the special needs child in learning centers. *Day Care and Early Education, Vol,* 43–44.

Jensema, C. J. (1994). Telecommunications for the deaf—Echoes of the past—a glimpse of the future. *American Annals of the Deaf, 139,* 22–27.

Kinney, P., Ouellette, T., & Wolery, M. (1989). Screening and assessing sensory functioning. In D. B. Bailey, Jr. & M. Wolery (Eds.), *Assessing infants and preschoolers with handicaps* (pp. 144–165). Columbus, OH: Merrill.

Kretschmer, R. R., & Messenheimer-Young, T. (1994). Can I play? A hearing-impaired preschooler requests to access maintained social interaction. *Volta Review, 96*(2), 5–17.

Ling, D. (1990). Advances underlying spoken language development: A century of building on Bell. *Volta Review, 42*(4), 8–17.

Luckner, J. (1991a). Mainstreaming hearing-impaired students: Perceptions of regular educators. *American-Speech-Language-Hearing Association, Vol* 302–305.

Luckner, J. (1991b). The competencies needed for teaching hearing impaired students. *American Annals of the Deaf, 136*(1), 17–20.

Luetke-Stahlman, B. (1998). Providing the support services needed by students who are deaf or hard of hearing. *American Annals of the Deaf, 143*(5), 338–391.

Martin, F. N. (1997). *Introduction to audiology: A review manual* (4th ed.). Boston: Allyn & Bacon.

Martin, F. N., & Noble, B. (1994). Hearing and hearing disorders. In G. Shames, E. Wiig, and W. Secord (Eds), *Human communication disorders: An introduction* (4th ed., pp. 388–436). New York: Merrill.

McArthur, S. H. (1982). *Raising your hearing impaired child: A guideline for parents.* Washington, DC: Alexander Graham Bell Association for the Deaf.

McCollister, F. P., Simpson, L. C., Dahle, A. J., Pass, R. F., Fowler, K. B., Amos, C. S., & Boll, T. J. (1996). Hearing loss and congenital symptomatic cytomegalovirus infection: A case report of multidisciplinary longitudinal assessment and intervention. *Journal of the American Academy of Audiology, 2,* 57–62.

Meadow-Orlans, K., Sass-Lehrer, M., Scott-Olson, K., & Mertens, D. (1998, January/February). Children who are hard of hearing: Are they forgotten? *Perspectives in Education and Deafness, 16*(3), 6–9.

Moestick, S. (1998). Opening doors for families of children who are deaf or hard of hearing. *The School Counselor, 51*(7), 70.

Mullis, F., & Otwell, P. (1998). Consulting with classroom teachers of students who are hearing impaired: Useful information for school counselors. *Journal of Humanistic Education and Development, 36*(4), 222–233.

Northern, J., & Downs, M. (1989). *Hearing in children.* Baltimore: Williams & Wilkins.

Northern, J., & Lemme, M. (1986). Hearing and auditory disorders. In G. Shames & E. Wiig (Eds.), *Human communication disorders* (p. 418). Columbus, OH: Merrill.

Nussbaum, D. (1988). *There's a hearing impaired child in my class.* Washington, DC: Gallaudet University.

O'Donoghue, G. (1999). Hearing without ears: Do cochlear implants work in children. *British Medical Journal, 318*(7176), 72–74.

Perigoe, C. (1992). Strategies for the remediation of speech-impaired children. *Volta Review, 94*(3), 95–111.

Quigley, S. P., & Kretschmer, R. E. (1982). *The education of deaf children.* Baltimore: University Park Press.

Seikel, J. S., King, D. W., & Drumright, D. G. (1997). *Anatomy and physiology for speech and language.* San Diego: Singular Publishing Group.

Skinner, P. (1985). Hearing. In P. Skinner & R. Shelton (Eds.), *Speech, language, and hearing: Normal processes and disorders* (2nd ed., pp. 170–191). New York: John Wiley & Sons.

Skinner, P., & Shelton. R. (1985). *Speech, language, and hearing: Normal processes and disorders* (2nd ed.). New York: John Wiley & Sons.

Smith, T., Polloway, E., Patton, J., & Dowdy, C. (1995). *Teaching students with special needs in inclusive settings.* Boston: Allyn & Bacon.

Stuckless, E. R., & Birch, S. W. (1997). The influence of early manual communication on the linguistic development of deaf children. *American Annals of the Deaf, 142*(3), 71–78.

Thomas, P., & Carmack, F. (1990). *Speech and language: Detecting and correcting special needs.* Boston: Allyn & Bacon.

U. S. Department of Health & Human Services. (1997, November 14). Serious hearing impairments among children aged 3–10 years. Atlanta, GA, 1991–1993. *Morbidity and Mortality Weekly Report, 46–45,* 1073–1074.

Van Riper, C. (1994). Audiology in 1936. *ASHA, 36,* 37.

Van Riper, C., & Erickson, R. (1996). *Speech correction. An introduction to speech pathology and audiology* (9th ed.). Boston: Allyn & Bacon.

Weiss, C., & Lillywhite, H. (1981). *Communication disorders: Prevention and early intervention.* St. Louis: C. V. Mosby.

Whitaker, M. (1998). Universal newborn hearing screening: It's on its way. *Hearing Journal, 51,* 21–28, 69.

Wilson, D. L. (1992, July 15). Dramatic breakthroughs for deaf students: New technologies offer greater participation. *Chronicle of Higher Education, Vol* 16–17.

10

Special Populations

Martha S. Lue

Chapter Objectives _____

On completion of this chapter, the reader will be able to:

- Identify common special populations and related communication disorders and syndromes; and
- Describe strategies that the classroom teacher might employ in working with these youngsters in regular, special, and inclusive settings.

- Seven-year-old Jeralyn is autistic. She has a younger sister and an older brother. She wears glasses and walks on her toes. Although the cause of her autism is unknown, genetic testing indicates that she has a chromosomal translocation. The testing revealed part of her fifth chromosome detached and reattached to the first chromosome.

  Currently, she has few verbal skills. Her parents use picture boards to assist her in communicating. When she is physically hurt, however, she does say the word *mom*. Her mother reports that when Jeralyn was four years old, she did have a ten- to fifteen-word speaking vocabulary, but it faded for no explained reason, and now she rarely speaks. She attends public school and spends fifteen minutes in the morning in a regular education class. The rest of the day is spent in a special education classroom. She sees a speech-language pathologist twice a week, but her teachers are less concerned with communication than with her daily living skills, such as toilet training and drinking from a cup with minimal spillage. At school, she uses an assistive technology device, Wolf, and similar assistive technology devices. (Assistive technology is discussed in Chapter 11).

- Julie is the mother of three girls, ages 6½ years, 5 years, and 9 months. The youngest, Shelby, has Down syndrome. Down syndrome is a chromosomal disorder characterized by mental retardation in most cases and physical signs such as slanted-appearing eyes, short stature, and flattened facial features. Shelby has been enrolled in an early intervention program since she was two weeks old. Part of Shelby's program includes bimonthly visits with a speech therapist and bimonthly visits with an occupational therapist, who also acts as a physical therapist. Shelby has well-developed social skills and her vocabulary is quite large, although a number of her words are hard to understand to people unfamiliar with her speech patterns. Due to fluid in her ears, Shelby hears as though she is underwater, a condition her mother reports will be rectified by tubes being placed in her ears. Her communication skills are positively reinforced by her parents and her two older sisters, who her mother says are great teachers and role models.

  In addition to Shelby's early intervention program, a student from the local university's exceptional education teacher training department works with her two to three times a week for a total of two hours. Julie, the mother, provides the student with certain play methods that are developmentally beneficial to Shelby. Julie is a member of a toy-lending group in which developmental toys may be checked out for short periods of time and returned. (Once the checked-out toys are returned, other toys may be checked out.)

- Barbara, the mother of three, recalled discovering, in the twenty-fourth week of pregnancy with one of her children, that the child would be born with a cleft lip and palate. To check for further abnormalities, an amniocentesis was performed. No other abnormalities were detected. When the child was born, a unilateral cleft lip and palate were present. (A cleft lip is a congenital splitting of the upper lip. A cleft palate is a congenital splitting of the middle of the palate.)

  Feeding problems were an immediate challenge. A special bottle with a special nipple was recommended and used. Surgery of the lip was performed at three months. The opening to the palate was closed at nine months. Tubes were also placed in the child's ears due to frequent ear infections.

  The child is now seven years of age, enrolled in a general education classroom, and attends speech therapy twice a week. Barbara has information on support groups, but has not felt she has needed to attend. The child will need additional surgery for further corrections and then further speech therapy.

Jeralyn and Shelby present syndromes that are now being seen more in inclusive settings. As more and more children with special needs are educated in more diverse and inclusive settings, special educators are assuming a more prominent role in working with youngsters and their families with various speech, language, and/or intellectual impairments. While all of these youngsters may not require the direct services of the speech-language pathologist, it is the special educator who will need additional knowledge regarding the problem, causation, and implications. Children may present symptoms from among conditions such as cerebral palsy, aphasia, Down syndrome, Prader-Willi syndrome, Hunter's syndrome, cleft lip and palate, Tourette syndrome, failure to thrive, prenatal alcohol syndrome (PAS), fetal alcohol syndrome (FAS), and autism. Parents of these children, as in the case of Barbara, may also be looking for answers and support in parenting from the classroom teacher, rather than from other parents of children with similar disabilities.

This chapter seeks to explore communication problems of various special populations—students who exhibit various syndromes or characteristics in classrooms, and the strategies that the special educator can use in meeting the needs of these students. (Students assessed as learning disabled, mentally disabled, and emotionally disabled will be discussed in another chapter.)

Syndromes and Communication Problems

The word *syndrome,* in a generic sense, refers to a group of symptoms that constitute a particular condition. Chermak and Wagner-Bitz (1993), discussing clinical genetics, cite work by Emery and Rimoin (1983) indicating that 1 in 50 infants is born with a major congenital abnormality. Further, there are at least 150 syndromes accompanying cleft palate, 198 syndromes associated with mental retardation, and 105 syndromes involving communication disorders secondary to structural anomalies of the ear, oral cavity, and brain.

Activity

Review and annotate three articles related to some communication problems that children with special needs exhibit. Compare and contrast important points, strategies, and perspectives.

Cerebral Palsy

Cerebral palsy (CP) refers to a group of disabling conditions caused by damage to the central nervous system. *Cerebral* refers to the brain or an area of the brain

(Vergason & Anderegg, 1997), while *palsy* describes lack of muscle control that is often the result of a nervous system dysfunction. Damage to the brain can occur pre-, peri-, or postnatally. Such damage may result from problems during the pregnancy, such as lack of oxygen to the fetus, from an illness during the pregnancy, from a premature delivery, or from a difficult delivery. Damage to the brain may occur early in life as a result of an accident, lead poisoning, illness, child abuse, or other factors.

CP is often referred to as a multidimensional, nonprogressive disorder that is a result of a central nervous system (CNS) injury that occurs during the early period of brain development (Bishop, Gyers-Brown, & Robson, 1990). While the damage may be nonprogressive, the effect of the damage can create more problems as further development or maturation occurs.

Incidence.   Out of every 5,000 Americans, sixteen have some degree of cerebral palsy. The National Information Center for Handicapped Children and Youth with Disabilities (1995) reports that 10,000 babies with cerebral palsy are born each year, while another 2,000 acquire it in the early years of life. Further, a report by the *New England Journal of Medicine* indicated that 100,000 Americans under the age of eighteen have some degree of neurologic disability attributable to cerebral palsy. Of that number, approximately 25 percent are unable to walk and 30 percent are classified as mentally disabled. One third of all children with cerebral palsy have epilepsy, and one half have hemiplegia (Kuban & Leviton, 1994).

Characteristics.   Six main descriptions of cerebral palsy have been recognized:

- **Spastic:** The most common CP, characterized by tense, contracted muscles; also accompanied by persistent primitive reflexes and absence or delay of normal motor skills;
- **Athetoid:** Characterized by constant uncontrolled movements (the second most prevalent type);
- **Ataxia:** Characterized by poor sense of balance and depth perception and lack of muscle coordination;
- **Mixed:** A combination of the types of cerebral palsy in which two or more areas of development are involved;
- **Rigidity:** Characterized by constant tension of muscles, which results in spasticity; and,
- **Tremor:** Characterized by shakiness of limbs; atonia or hypertonia.

Accompanying/concomitant problems may include, but are not limited to, the following: seizures, problems in vision, hearing, or speech, abnormal sensation or perception, mental retardation, and impairments in arm and leg movement. Bear in mind that each case is different, and that some individuals who have cerebral palsy may have no associated medical disorders (National Institute of Neurological Disorders and Stroke, 1996).

Etiology Related to Cerebral Palsy.   While etiologies vary, the most frequently cited causes in the literature include: anoxia, prenatal factors, mother–baby blood type incompatibilities, toxins, prematurity, genetic syndromes, chromosomal abnormalities, preeclampsia, sepsis, asphyxia, and traumatic brain injury. The majority of cases of cerebral palsy originate during intrauterine development (Friedman & Weiss, 1991). While some researchers suggest that anoxia is the primary cause of cerebral palsy, Baker (1991) asserts that 78 percent of the children with cerebral palsy have not suffered anoxia at birth. The majority of babies with cerebral palsy, he adds, develop this disorder during the first trimester of pregnancy.

Cognitive Development.   A wide range of intellectual capabilities exist among children with cerebral palsy. Cognitive development will vary depending on the extent and place of injury to the brain (Shiminiski-Maher, 1989). While some youngsters who have cerebral palsy may have severely impaired cognitive development, others may have IQs that fall in the range of gifted (Willard-Holt, 1998). In other words, the same range of ability may occur in people with CP as is found in normal populations.

Speech Development.   As learned in previous chapters, speech production involves the respiratory system. Some youngsters with cerebral palsy do not have enough respiratory control to develop intelligible speech. Irregular breathing affects vocal production, which is revealed in the child's problems in sustaining and varying vocal production. Children lacking respiratory control may talk in a quiet, whispered voice or they might have outbursts of loud, uncontrolled sounds. If a child is unable to sustain voice production, his or her length of utterance may be restricted, even though the child may be cognitively aware of syntactic structures and be capable of cognitively producing sentences (Peterson, 1987).

Educational Implications of Working with a Child with Cerebral Palsy.
Treatment of an individual with cerebral palsy requires a multidisciplinary team approach. Team members may include parents, educators, medical personnel, social services personnel, speech pathologists, and the individual. The team members' task should be to provide the most appropriate and optimal learning environment for the child.

To promote social-emotional growth, parents, teachers, and classmates should avoid overprotection and encourage children to take risks within the limits of safety. Teachers and classmates should be cognizant of the fact that although children with cerebral palsy may be physically disabled, these youngsters are more like their classmates than different from them. Some factors that can help facilitate communication include: early consultation with a speech-language pathologist, encouraging breathing/control exercises (if appropriate), using concrete articles and pictures to reinforce speech, and employing feeding techniques that help to facilitate speech.

Aphasia

A language disorder caused by brain damage due to either stroke or trauma is covered by the term *aphasia.* Moreover, aphasia is a multiple-modality loss of language ability, usually caused by damage to the dominant hemisphere of the brain (Gary & Jermier, 1988). Usually all modes of language usage are impaired to some degree. The mode may include speaking, understanding, reading, writing, and gesturing. Aphasia interferes with one's ability to use language, to share one's thoughts, and/or to understand the expressions of others.

Specific speech/language/neuromuscular problems related to aphasia include:

- Apraxia: A neurologically based articulation disorder that involves an inability to make articulatory movements, even though involuntary and voluntary movements of the speech mechanisms occur normally. The apraxic individual may use the mouth normally for swallowing, but may make articulatory errors. These errors are likely to involve sound repetitions, additions, and substitutions of some sounds for others. Individuals appear to repeat and struggle with words, although comprehension may not be affected.
- Dysarthria: A slurred, uncoordinated, and imprecise speech due to motor dysfunctions. Speech may be hypernasal and voice breathy or harsh, slow or choppy, or monotone.

Down Syndrome

One of the most widely recognized types of mental retardation, **Down syndrome** is thought to be caused by a chromosomal abnormality. Chromosomal abnormalities may occur when there are aberrations in chromosomal arrangements, either before fertilization or during early cell division (Hardman, Drew, & Egan, 1999). It is believed that in individuals with Down syndrome, an extra partial or complete twenty-first chromosome results in the characteristics. Chromosomes are thread-like structures composed of DNA and other proteins. Human cells normally have 46 chromosomes. They are paired off in 23. In Down syndrome, 95 percent of all cases are reported to be caused by the event of one cell having 21 chromosomes instead of one. This results in the fertilized egg having three twenty-first chromosomes (Leshin, 1997–1998). In a few cases, the extra chromosome 21 is attached to another chromosome in the egg or sperm, creating a condition called *Translocation Down syndrome.*

It has been estimated that nearly 4,000 infants, or 1 in every 1000 live births in the United States, are born with Down syndrome (National Information Center for Children and Youth with Disabilities, 1991). For mothers between the ages of twenty and thirty, the chance of having a child born with Down syndrome is 1 in 1200 (MacMillan, 1982). Abroms and Bennett (1983) add that in about 25 percent of youngsters born with a specific type of Down syndrome, Trisomy 21 (the most common type of Down syndrome), the age of the father (particularly when the father is over 55 years of age) appears to be a factor.

Characteristics. More than fifty traits have been identified with Down syndrome (Howard, Williams, Port, & Lepper, 1997). Not all individuals with Down syndrome share the same physical characteristics. However, the most distinguishing physical and mental traits of Down syndrome include:

- low muscle tone (muscle hypotonia);
- some degree of mental retardation in a majority of cases;
- flat facial profile, including a depressed nasal bridge and small nose (caused by underdevelopment of the nasal bone);
- upward slant to the eyes;
- abnormal shape and small size of the ears;
- single deep crease across the center of the palm;
- excessive ability to extend the joints;
- fifth finger has one bending joint instead of two;
- small skin folds on the inner corner of the eyes;
- excessive space between large and second toe;
- short, stocky build;
- high incidence of hearing impairments with a tendency toward high-frequency hearing losses;
- delayed motor and speech development; and
- enlargement of tongue in relationship to size of the mouth (National Down Syndrome Society, n.d.; Drew, Hardman, & Logan, 1996).

Additionally, it is believed that half of the children born with Down syndrome have congenital heart defects. Further, these youngsters appear to have increased susceptibility to infection, respiratory problems, and obstructed digestive tracts. Associated illnesses or diseases may include Hirschsprung's disease, hypothyroidism, and epilepsy (Leshin, 1997–1998).

Educational Implications. Children with Down syndrome are educated in a variety of educational settings, depending on the nature and severity of the disability, and the recommendations made by the members of the IEP team. The following are general recommendations that need to be considered:

- Early intervention for children and their families is essential. Most school districts now have in place teams of early childhood education professionals that work with children and their families;
- Parents should be encouraged to join support groups, such as the National Down Syndrome Society. Many support groups have a national toll-free number that provides information about local affiliations, conferences, ongoing research, and so forth;

- Intervention goals should include emphasis on motor and language development. Therapists and educators in early intervention programs can teach parents how to help their babies to develop skills in gross and fine motor, language, social development, and self-help;
- With early intervention and specialized services, many children with Down syndrome can be fully integrated in the regular classroom.

Further, it has been reported that as children with Down syndrome grow older, their relative intellectual abilities diminish compared to the rate of progress made by typical children (Rynders & Horrobin, 1990). The National Down Syndrome Society (n.d.) reports that adults with Down syndrome are at increased risk for Alzheimer's disease. In the general population, approximately 6 percent will develop Alzheimer's. For individuals with Down syndrome, that number grows to 25 percent.

Prader-Willi Syndrome

Prader-Willi syndrome (PWS) was initially reported in 1956. It is a chromosomal disorder that is estimated to occur once in every 10,000 births. The syndrome results in muscular hypotonia, obesity, short stature, hypogonadism, and, frequently, some degree of cognitive dysfunction. After an initial period of poor growth, children with Prader-Willi syndrome may gain weight rapidly, usually between the ages of one and four years (Crnic, Sulzbacher, & Holm, 1980). Associated characteristics may include:

- Delayed development of language (Dyson & Lombardino, 1989);
- Learning disabilities: Although many children with Prader-Willi syndrome have mental retardation, based on their tested IQ, their performances are more like those seen in children with learning disabilities in that there appears to be considerable variability in skills and deficits exhibited by each individual;
- General cognitive dysfunction; and,
- Impaired speech production, ranging from mild articulation distortions to speech intelligibility.

Other facts about Prader-Willi include:

- a slightly higher prevalence rate in boys; and,
- a potential higher recurrence risk factor within some families who have had a child with Prader-Willi syndrome.

A precise etiology of the syndrome has not yet been established to apply to all cases. About 50 percent of people with Prader-Willi syndrome demonstrate some form of chromosome 15 abnormality (Kleppe, Katayana, Shipley, & Foushee, 1990). The syndrome may also be associated with a hypothalamic defect, which may account for the appetite control difficulties and emotional lability. Bierne-Smith, It-tenbach, and Patton (1998) add that the child with Prader-Willi syndrome has a preoccupation with eating that may prompt others to comment that for a child with this syndrome, life is viewed as "an endless meal" (p. 155).

Speech-Language Characteristics.   There are major speech and language characteristics that are associated with Prader-Willi:

- Delayed speech and articulation development;
- A high, narrow palatal arch;
- Micrognathia; and
- Inadequate velopharyngeal movement/closure.

Educational Implications for the Classroom Teacher.   The Prader-Willi Syndrome Association (1998) offers the following strategies for classroom management and general activities in working with individuals with this syndrome:

- Adapting to change may be very difficult for this child. A degree of consistency, predictability, and sameness in routine may be helpful;
- Make sure that all people involved with the child are aware of the need for dietary control required by these children;
- Encourage the development of social skills such as standing at an appropriate distance when communicating, taking turns in communicating, and sharing;
- Use humor to defuse potentially explosive situations;
- Encourage physical exercise with these children to the extent possible;
- Agree with other members of the collaborative team on steps taken to deal with inappropriate behaviors and be consistent with the guidelines that the team has initiated; and
- Involvement of parents is critical. Collaborative input on how the child is being managed is essential. All involved should agree on the strategies that apply, whether at school or at another setting.

Hunter's Syndrome

Hunter's syndrome, a genetic disorder, affects a very small percentage of the population. It is a result of enzymes that function improperly, which in turn cause a variety of functions in the body to change. It progresses as the child becomes older.
Facial characteristics may include:

- full cheeks
- thick lips
- protruding jaw
- short neck
- larger than normal head

- shortness
- hairiness
- protruding abdomen
- progressive hearing loss
- speech and language problems with structural changes within the vocal organs
- pulmonary abnormalities

At present, there are few available data on incidence. One statistic from Great Britain puts its incidence at 1 in 171,132 live births. In mild cases, the life span is 21.7 years. When death occurs, it is usually due to cardiac problems. In severe form, the average life span is 11.77 years.

Activity

Review research related to "orphan syndromes" or syndromes with a low incidence rate, but ones that may be seen in some classrooms. Report your findings to the class.

Cleft Lip and Palate

A cleft is an opening in the lip, the roof of the mouth (hard palate), or the soft tissue in the back of the mouth (soft palate). In some cases, this may include the bone of the upper jaw. More specifically, a **cleft palate** is an opening in the roof of the mouth (hard palate) in which the two sides of the palate did not join together.

Why Clefts Occur.   The human face develops during the first eight to ten weeks of gestation. If there is a disruption in development at some point between the sixth and eleventh weeks, a cleft may result. Fusion of the palate takes place from the front to the back of the mouth. Any disruption in this process will result in a palatal cleft. The earlier the interruption occurs, the more extensive the cleft will be. Congenital defects such as cleft lips and palates occur approximately once in every 600 to 1,200 births.

Additionally, clefts vary in their occurrence rate from one racial group to another. For example, Asians have the highest rate, 1 in 500. In Caucasians, the rate varies from 1 in 750 to 1 in 1,000 births. Clefts affect more boys than girls. One quarter of persons with clefts have cleft lips, one quarter have cleft palate, and half have both (Levine, 1990). There are at least one hundred syndromes associated with clefting.

Types of Clefts.   Types of clefts include unilateral or bilateral cleft of the lip and palate. In unilateral cleft of the lip and palate, the **premaxilla** and the **maxilla** fuse on one side only as do the bones of the hard palate and the nasal septum. This condition may be associated with a cleft of the palate or may exist as the only malformation (Moran & Pentz, 1995). Bilateral cleft of the lip and palate occur when neither side of the premaxilla, the maxilla, or the palatal bones fuse together. Other clefts may include: the hard palate only; the soft palate only; both the hard and soft palate; and clefts of the lip only. Clefts of the lip may vary as little as the border of the lip or the cleft may extend upward and into the nostril. Submucous cleft is a condition in which the muscles of the soft palate have failed to unite at the midline, but the mucousal membrane has fused to hide the underlying cleft. Figure 10.1 presents both normal and cleft palate configurations.

    Clefts are repaired surgically. The lip is typically repaired early in the first year of life. Surgical repair of the palate is most commonly done before two years of age, with additional surgeries as needed. Clefting may interfere with swallowing and breathing, as well as with appearance and proper sound formation. Infections may result also from serious lack of closure in the mouth and nasal area.

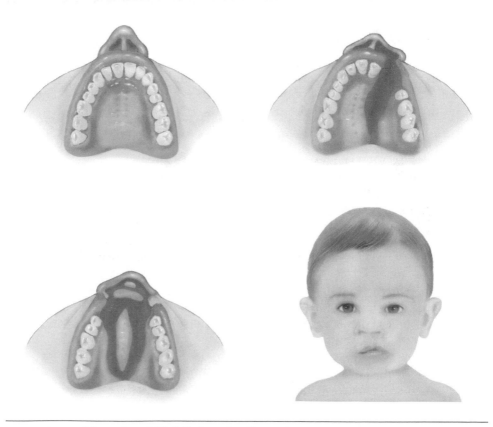

FIGURE 10.1 *Normal and Cleft Palate Configurations*

From M. L. Hardman, C. J. Drew, & M. W. Egan (1999). In *Human exceptionality. Society, school, and family* (6th ed., p. 316). Boston: Allyn & Bacon. Reprinted with permission.

Early Speech Development and Cleft Palate.   Through our understanding of normal speech production, we know that a cleft of the palate may affect speech because it prevents the complete separation at the oral and nasal regions (Moran & Pentz, 1995). Estrem and Broen (1989) compared the first fifty words produced by five children with no oral–facial abnormality and five children with cleft palate. As a group, children with cleft palates tended to target more words with initial nasals, approximates, and vowels and fewer words with word-initial stops, fricatives, and affricates.

Communication Problems Associated with Clefting.   Although most students with cleft lip or palate will have had the surgery done to repair the cleft before they enter school, some communication problems may remain:

- Language delay because of disruptions to communicative development;
- Hyponasality related to structural deviations of the nasal cavity and nasal septum;
- Hypernasality related to inadequate velopharyngeal closure;
- Consonant distortions caused by audible nasal air flow such as nasal snorting or snorting related to inadequate velopharyngeal closure;
- Delay in articulation development;
- Misarticulations related to hearing loss; and,
- Cosmetic distortions and other facial grimaces related to attempts at preventing nasal airflow.

Velopharyngeal Competence and Cleft Palate.   Normal speakers of English use the velum and pharyngeal muscles to close the passage between the oral and nasal cavities during the production of all sounds except nasal consonants. Failure to produce this velopharyngeal closure during speech sometimes affects vowels as they occur adjacent to nasal consonants. **Velopharyngeal closure** occurs when the velum (soft palate) and pharyngeal walls act together to direct air and voice through the mouth, rather than the nose. The inability to achieve total closure of the nasal cavity during speech is termed **velopharyngeal incompetence.**

Surgical Treatment for Cleft Lip/Cleft Palate.   Surgery is often used to correct the physical problems of cleft lip/palate and isolated cleft palate. The timing however, is dependent on a number of factors:

- preference of the individual surgeon;
- the general health of the baby; and,
- the nature of the cleft (March of Dimes Birth Defects Foundation, 1999).

Each child is different. Some children may require more surgeries than others. Figures found in the literature related to surgical repair include the following:

- Primary repair, at approximately ten weeks;
- Palatal repair, at approximately nine to twelve months;
- Secondary repair (if needed), at approximately four to six years;
- Alveolar cleft, at eight to ten years; and
- Final repair (if needed), at fourteen to sixteen years (Texas Pediatric Surgical Associates, n.d.).

Members of the Cleft Palate Interdisciplinary Team.   Many children with clefts experience special problems, especially in relationship to feeding, ear diseases, speech development, and dental problems. Many of these problems are related to each other in some way. In order to produce the best solution for managing cleft palate problems—physically, emotionally, and linguistically—an interdisciplinary team works together to provide options for necessary procedures.

The team may include:

- General surgeon—Surgery is usually performed at the age of ten weeks for cleft lip. Palate surgery is done at six to eight months.
- Otolaryngologist (Ear, Nose, and Throat Specialist)—Treats the condition medically or surgically.
- Pediatrician—A medical doctor who specializes in the general care of children.
- Orthodontist—A dentist with additional training. This discipline is concerned with the alignment of teeth and the correction of malocclusion.
- Prosthodontist—The dentist who is responsible for the construction and fitting of various dental appliances, such as dentures, obturators, and palatal devices.
- Pedodontist—A dentist who specializes in children's dental care and works with a team in overall management of the child's dental care.
- Speech-language pathologist—A trained individual at the master's or doctoral level who works with children and adults who have demonstrated communication problems.
- Audiologist—A nonmedical hearing specialist who tests for hearing sensitivity and administers diagnostic hearing tests to children and adults with suspected hearing loss and/or various hearing disorders.
- Plastic surgeon—A physician certified in plastic surgery who surgically repairs the cleft.
- Classroom teacher—Often observes children in the classroom who communicate poorly and refers them to the audiologist and/or speech-language pathologist, or works with children after diagnosis and recommended therapy.

Educational Implications for the Student with Cleft Lip/Palate.   Speech-language therapy is one of the most frequently provided related services for children with cleft lip/palate. Therefore, classroom teachers work very closely with the speech-language pathologist to ensure that the speech-language goals are being met in the classroom and are being infused in the child's academic in-class programs (Turnbull, Turnbull, Shank, & Leal, 1999).

The potential for failure to thrive because of a decreased ability to eat is also a significant problem for infants born with cleft palate. The multidisciplinary team throughout the school years will see many children with cleft lip/palate. In most cases, the speech-language pathologist will continue to work with these children in school settings. Keep in mind that most of these children will be educated in a regular education setting with classroom support, where needed.

Reed (1994) reminds us that nearly all children with cleft palate will have reduced speech intelligibility until the cleft has been surgically repaired and they are able to adjust to the changes in the speech mechanism. As a result, initially or during the first few years, there may be a gap in lexical acquisition, but as they grow older the gap in language abilities appears to close. However, problems remain related to interpersonal factors, such as concerns about personal appearance and acceptance.

Mastropieri and Scruggs (2000) add that it is the environment—an open, accepting one—that is most important in promoting acceptance and decreasing the opportunity for ridicule and anxiety. The classroom teacher may wish to speak privately to those students suspected of teasing and ridicule, and ask their help and support.

In cases where there is hearing loss, educational methods and strategies appropriate for youngsters with hearing impairments should be employed (Blackman, 1983). (For more specific suggestions in this area, the reader is referred to the chapter on Problems of Hearing: Identification and Remediation.)

Activity

Contact a professional in one of the specialties cited. Arrange for an interview to gain additional insight about the special populations discussed.

Specific suggestions by Moran and Pentz (1995) for helping children with cleft lip or palate include:

- Know what kinds of problems to suspect—the nature and severity of the articulation problem, and so forth;
- Be alert to possible problems of socialization;
- Be prepared to assist the student in making up work, due to illness, doctors' appointments, hospitalization, and so on.

The important thing to remember is that these children are *children* first. Each is different and unique. It is the classroom teacher who sets the tone for acceptance and support.

Tourette Syndrome

Tourette syndrome (TS) is a neurological disorder characterized by tics, involuntary, rapid, sudden movements that may occur repeatedly in the same way (American Psychiatric Association, 1994). Symptoms are multiple motor, with one or more vocal tics present at some time during the span of the illness. A *tic* is an involuntary, recurrent, brief twitching of a group of muscles (Dox, Melloni, & Eisner, 1985). The occurrence of tics may occur many times a day, nearly every day, or intermittently throughout a span of more than one year, with a periodic change in the number, frequency, type, and location of the tics, and in their sensitivity. The onset occurs before the age of twenty-one and continues through a normal lifespan. Males appear to be affected three to four times more often than females.

There are two categories of tics, simple and complex. These are further divided into two subcategories, motor and vocal. Simple motor tics include eye blinking, head jerking, shoulder shrugging, and facial grimacing; throat clearing, barking, sniffing, and tongue clicking are among the simple vocal tics. Complex motor tics include jumping, touching other people or things, smelling, twirling about, and self-injurious actions. Uttering ordinary words or phrases, **coprolalia,** swearing, vocalizing (and other socially unacceptable terms), and echolalia characterize complex vocal tics.

Associated Behavioral Problems. In addition to the behaviors previously described, individuals with Tourette syndrome may also exhibit the following behaviors:

- Obsessions (repetitive or bothersome thoughts);
- Compulsions and ritualistic behaviors;
- Attention deficit disorders (ADD) with or without hyperactivity; and
- Difficulties with impulse control.

Cognitive Development. This syndrome may occur in people with any level of intellectual function, and within a wide range of etiologies (Bodfish, Rosenquist, & Thompson, 1997). Nearly half may exhibit problems in at least one area of learning disability (Burd, Kauffman, & Kerbeshian, 1992). The areas may include reading, writing, math, and/or perceptual difficulties.

Educational Implications for the Classroom Teacher. Students identified as having Tourette syndrome have the same IQ range as the general population, but many exhibit some form of a learning disability. This problem, combined with the frequent tics and problems of attention, may render the individual eligible for special education assistance. The following strategies are helpful in both special and regular education settings (Tourette Syndrome Association, 1997; Knoblauch, 1998):

- Exhibit and model tolerance for the child's tics, movements, and noises;
- Provide opportunities for short breaks outside of the classroom so that the child can relax and release the tics;

- Allow the student the opportunity to take exams in a private room, so that the child can focus on the task at hand and not waste energy trying to suppress the tics;
- Assist other students in understanding the syndrome, and call on the school counselor, the child's parents, and/or a member from the Tourette Syndrome Association to provide information about the syndrome;
- Seat the child in front of you for all instructions and directions to minimize the visual distractions of classmates; and
- If tics are particularly disruptive, consider eliminating reciting in front of the class for a while; a tape recorder can be used for oral reports.

Table 10.1 contains additional information about Tourette syndrome.

Failure to Thrive

Failure to thrive, in a broad sense, describes the failure of growth and development in infants, toddlers, school-age children, and adolescents to meet realistic expectations. This may be due, in part, to genetic, physical, psychological, or social factors. These are youngsters who weigh significantly less than their peers or who gain weight at a slower than normal rate during infancy or early childhood. Infants and children who fall at least two standard deviations below the norm over a designated time period (Howard, Williams, Port, & Lepper, 1997) may be considered to be "failing to thrive."

TABLE 10.1   *Tourette Syndrome at a Glance*

- It is a neurological impairment that may be triggered by stress.
- One in 200 children in the United States has Tourette syndrome, as reported by the National Institutes of Health.
- These youngsters act normally most of the time, but suddenly they may twitch, blurt out ridiculous words, swear, scream, kick a wall, or punch.
- Reactions appear to occur from a chemical imbalance in the brain, rather than being willful behavior, as they are often perceived to be.
- The Tourette Syndrome Association reports that up to 90 percent of people with Tourette Syndrome never see a doctor or seek treatment.
- Once a rage has hit in those with Tourette syndrome, wait until it passes; then discuss the matter with the child. Tourette's ruins lives. (Orlando Sentinel, 1998, December 6, A-25.)
- When Tourette syndrome is accompanied by other disorders, such as attention deficit hyperactivity disorder and obsessive compulsive disorder, it is called *Tourette's Plus*.
- The Tourette Syndrome Association is located in Bayside, NY.

Possible causes may include, but are not limited to:

- Chromosomal abnormalities (Down syndrome and Turner syndrome);
- Abnormalities of the endocrine syndrome; and
- Inadequate economic means.

Causes may stem from inappropriate dietary and feeding practices, environmental stress, emotional stress, abuse, and neglect. Children may also have reduced abilities in language, attention, and memory.

Prenatal Alcohol Syndrome (PAS)/Fetal Alcohol Syndrome

Fetal alcohol syndrome (FAS) is now recognized as the leading known preventable cause of mental retardation in the United States. It is reported to occur in 1 out of every 750 live births. In some Native American populations, the incidence of FAS has been reported to be up to 10 times higher (Abkarian, 1992). Research appears to suggest that even moderate maternal alcohol consumption may be linked to a variety of developmental and school-related difficulties. For mothers who abuse alcohol chronically, fetal alcohol syndrome live births are reported to average 71 per 1,000 (Abel, 1990). Further, there is some evidence to suggest that offspring of certain groups may be at considerable risk for fetal alcohol syndrome. The highest incidence rates of FAS (19.5 per 1,000) have been reported among the Apache and Ute tribes of the American Southwest and the Canadian Indians of British Colombia (Phelps & Grabowski, 1992).

Babies born with fetal alcohol syndrome generally have a low birth weight of less than 2,500 grams or 5.5 pounds. These babies also suffer from prenatal and postnatal growth deficiencies. That is, they have a linear growth rate of only about 65 percent that of normal children, and a weight rate of about 40 percent less than normal. They show early signs of mental retardation, with IQ's in the mild to moderate ranges, accompanied by frequent microcephalia (Phelps & Grabowski, 1992),

Babies with fetal alcohol syndrome may suffer from distortion of facial features, narrow eyelids, a sunken nasal bridge that gives a flat face appearance, drooping eyelids, and very thin lips.

Deformities in body organs and other structures depend on when the damage occurred. Damage can result in malformed legs, defective body organs, as well as a frequent occurrence of heart defects. As these children grow in years, behavior problems may often be seen as hyperactivity or "extreme nervousness" and poor attention span.

Language Development.   Extreme deficits in both receptive and expressive language skills have been reported (Arnold, Johnson, Madison, Schulthis, & Seikel, 1998). Characteristics may also include delayed use of sentences or more complex grammatical units, inadequate comprehension, and problems in short term memory (Phelps & Grabowski, 1992).

Characteristics of the Substance Exposed Infant.   Infants who are exposed to alcohol and other drugs while being carried by their mothers have an increased risk of suffering from physical, emotional, and social abnormalities that can include, but are not limited to:

Physical
- low birth weight
- small head circumference
- impaired motor development
- abnormally formed internal organs
- irregular sleeping patterns
- poor feeding patterns
- hypertonicity/hypotonicity

They often exhibit symptoms similar to those of adults using or withdrawing from drugs.

Emotional
- irritability
- frequent startles
- unresponsiveness
- difficulty with being comforted or consoling self
- frequent gaze aversion
- poor interactive capacities

Educational Implications for Substance Exposed Infants and Children.   Children prenatally exposed to drugs may face serious educational challenges. It then becomes your role as a classroom teacher to develop strategies that will assist the child in developing to his or her maximum potential. The ERIC Clearinghouse on Disabilities and Gifted Education (Pinkerton, 1991) is an excellent place to start in developing your professional library on strategies that you might employ in working effectively with this child.

- Curricula should be developmentally appropriate and promote experiential learning, exploration, interaction, and play in an interesting and relevant context;
- Continuous assessment should be done by the teacher or primary caregiver in a number of settings and instructional arrangements—during play, during transition, and so on;
- A flexible room environment that allows materials and equipment to be removed to reduce stimuli or added to enrich the environment should be provided; and
- Recognize the child's strengths and the ways in which she or he is a typical child.

Autism

The word *autism* is taken from the Greek *autos,* meaning "self," to indicate the extreme sense of isolation and detachment from the world that characterizes some individuals with autism (Hardman, Drew, & Egan, 1999). The syndrome became a recognized disability category with the passing of the Individuals with Disabilities Education Act in 1990.

Autism is a developmental disorder, with severe distortions of social and language development, that begins at an early age. Individuals with autism may demonstrate a number of unusual behaviors and characteristics:

- Impaired social relationships;
- Lack of responsiveness to other people;
- Grossly impaired development of language;
- Unusual speech patterns, when speech is present, such as echolalia;
- Bizarre interactions with, or responses to, the environment, such as extreme fascination with unusual objects, resistance to even minor changes, and behavior rituals (often involving repetitive acts such as flicking the fingers), which, if interfered with, lead to great distress or tantrums; and
- Self-injurious behavior.

Autism appears in approximately one child per 2,000 and appears to be more common in boys. Half of the autistic population never develops communication skills, while others exhibit echolalia. Further, the majority of individuals with autism show other abnormal speech patterns (Schubert, 1997).

Educational Implications.   When developing an educational plan for the child with autism, bear in mind that each child is different and has varying levels of abilities and disabilities. Keep in mind that the plan for this child, as with other children with special needs, will need to be individualized and based on the unique needs of the student. As you develop this plan to maximize the child's learning potential, do not forget to involve all members of the collaborative team—parents, speech language professionals, school psychologists, behavioral specialists, and other individuals that you deem appropriate. The following are some generic strategies that you can employ (Saskatchewan Special Education Unit, 1998):

- Assist the student in learning acceptable limits;
- Give the student control within a structured situation;
- Be aware that the student may attempt to relate through negative behavior;
- To the extent appropriate, use visual methods of teaching;
- Provide a structured, predictable classroom environment;
- Use meaningful reinforcements;
- Use concrete examples and hands-on activities;
- Avoid long strings of verbal information;
- Identify tasks and activities that tend to create frustration for the child;

- Plan for transitions and inform the student when the transition will occur;
- Provide opportunities for meaningful contact with the student's peers; and
- Set up communication opportunities to encourage expression.

Intervention and Treatments.   Approaches for treatment include focusing on specific observable behaviors and therapies focused on causation (Wehman, 1992). Educational interventions include instructional options ranging from specialized programs to integrated placement with support services.

Many significant shifts in the education of young children with autism have been noted. Many may require one-to-one instruction, while others may benefit from small group instruction. For specific strategies in working with both nonverbal and verbal students with autism, readers are referred to Layton and Watson (1995) and Twachtman (1995).

Including Students in General Education Settings.   As we continue to move toward including students with disabilities in general education settings, issues such as physical classroom space, class members' attitudes, and peers' social responses must be addressed (Clark & Smith, 1999). This effort requires commitment, support, and preparation by special and general education teachers, as well as from families and peers.

> ### Activity
>
> **Invite a member of a support group of parents of special needs children to your class.**

Summary

"Not all children" notes Ratner (1997), "acquire language easily and well" (p. 348). Communication and language problems are found in all groups of students—those with or without disabilities. In this chapter, I have attempted to describe some communication problems commonly found in some special populations. Characteristics, cognitive and language development, and educational implications were also examined. A brief orientation to specific disabilities/syndromes, identifying characteristics, language and communication characteristics, and educational implications for the general and special educator were included.

Keep in mind that students with communication, language, and speech problems are just as diverse as their abilities or disabilities. Many strategies that you have learned in working with other populations will certainly be effective in working with these youngsters. While no one chapter can possibly describe all of the different syndromes or disabilities that might be found in inclusive settings, it is hoped that the information presented will generate or spark interest in the unique needs and abilities of these students.

References and Suggested Readings

Abel, E. L. (1990). *Fetal alcohol syndrome*. Oradel, NJ: Medical Economics Books.

Abkarian, G. G. (1992). Communication effects of prenatal alcohol exposure. *Journal of Communication Disorders, 25,* 221–235.

Abroms, K. L., & Bennett, J. W. (1983). Current findings in Down's syndrome. *Exceptional Children, 49,* 449–450.

Adkins, E. (1991). Nursing care of clients with impaired communication. *Rehabilitation Nursing, 16*(2), 74–75.

Allessandri, M., Fuentes, F., Handelman, J. S., Harris, S. L., & Kristoff, B. (1991). A specialized program for preschool children with autism. *Language, Speech and Hearing Services in the Schools, 22*(3), 107–110.

Alporn, C. (1992). Hunter's syndrome and its management in a public school setting. *Language, Speech, and Hearing Services in the Schools, 23,* 102–106.

American Psychiatric Association. (1994). *Diagnostic and statistical manual of mental disorders* (4th ed.). Washington, DC: Author.

Arnold, M., Johnson, J., Madison, C. L., Schulthis, L., & Seikel, J. A. (1998). Comparative study of the phonology of preschool children prenatally exposed to cocaine and multiple drugs and non-exposed children. *Journal of Communication Disorders, 31*(3), 231–243.

Baker, S. (1991). Cerebral palsy: Trauma in the womb. *Health, 23,* 20.

Berecz, J. M. (1992). *Understanding Tourette syndrome, obsessive compulsive disorders, and related problems.* New York: Springer.

Bierne-Smith, M., Ittenbach, R., & Patton, J. (1998). *Mental retardation* (5th ed.). Upper Saddle River, NJ: Prentice-Hall.

Bigg, J. L. (1982). *Teaching individuals with physical and multiple disabilities.* New York: Charles E. Merrill.

Bishop, D. V., Gyers-Brown, B., & Robson, J. (1990). The relationship between phoneme discrimination, speech production, and language comprehension in cerebral-palsied individuals. *Journal of Speech and Hearing Research, 33*(2), 210–219.

Blackman, J. A. (1983). *Medical aspects of developmental disabilities in children birth to three: A resource for special-service providers in the educational setting.* Iowa City, IA: University of Iowa, Division of Developmental Disabilities.

Bodfish, J., Rosenquist, P., & Thompson, R. (1997). Tourette syndrome associated with mental retardation: A single-subject treatment study with haloperidol. *American Journal on Mental Retardation, 10*(5), 497–504.

Bronheim, S. (1991). An educator's guide to Tourette syndrome. *Journal of Learning Disabilities, 24,* 17–22.

Burd, L., Kauffman, D. W., & Kerbeshian, J. (1992). Tourette syndrome and learning disabilities. *Journal of Learning Disabilities, 25,* 598–604.

Chermak, G., & Wagner-Bitz, C. (1993). Survey of speech-language pathologists' and audiologists' knowledge of clinical genetics. *ASHA Journal, 35*(5), 31–45.

Clark, D., & Smith, S. (1999). Facilitating friendships: Including students with autism in the early elementary classroom. *Intervention in School and Clinic, 34*(4), 248–250.

Cohen, D. J., Brunin, R. D., & Teckman, J. (1988). *Tourette Syndrome and Tic disorders: Crucial understanding and treatment.* New York: John Wiley & Sons.

Cristoff, K., & Kane, S. (1991). Relationship building for students with autism. *TEACHING Exceptional Children, 23*(2), 49–51.

Crnic, K., Sulzbacher, S., & Holm, V. (1980). Preventing mental retardation associated with obesity in the Prader-Willi syndrome. *Pediatrics, 66*(5), 787–789.

Deisenberg, A., Murkoff, H., & Hathaway, S. (1988). *What to expect the first year.* New York: Workman.

Dox, I., Melloni, B. J., & Eisner, G. M. (1985). *Melloni's illustrated medical dictionary* (2nd ed.). Baltimore: Williams & Wilkins.

Drew, C. J., Hardman, M. L., & Logan, D. R. (1996). *Mental retardation: A life cycle approach* (4th ed.). Englewood Cliffs, NJ: Prentice-Hall.

Dyson, A., & Lombardino, L. (1989). Phonologic abilities of a preschool child with Prader-Willi syndrome. *Journal of Speech and Hearing Disorders, 54,* 44–48.

Emery, A. E. H., & Rimoin, D. L. (1983). Nature and incidence of genetic disease. In A. E. H. Emery & D. L. Rimoin (Eds), *Principles and practice of medical genetics* (pp. 1–4). New York: Churchill Livingstone.

Estrem, T., & Broen, P. (1989). Early speech production of children with cleft palate. *Journal of Speech and Hearing Research, 32,* 12–23.

Friedman, M., & Weiss, E. (1991). What you should know about cerebral palsy. *Parents Magazine, 66* (3), 68–74.

Gary, R., & Jermier, B. (1988). *Stroke: How to start the long road back. RN Journal, 49*(1), 49–54.

Hardman, M., Drew, C., & Egan, M. (1999). *Human exceptionality: Society, school, and family* (6th ed.). Boston: Allyn & Bacon.

Holm, V. (1981). The diagnosis of Prader-Willi Syndrome. In V. Holm, S. Sulzbacher, & P. L. Pipes (Eds.), *Prader-Willi syndrome* (pp. 45–53). Baltimore: University Park Press.

Howard, V. F., Williams, B. F., Port, P. D., & Lepper, C. (1997). *Very young children with special needs.* Upper Saddle River, NJ: Merrill/Prentice-Hall.

Huruitz, J., Picket, S. M., & Rilla, D.C. (1987). Promoting children's language interaction. *TEACHING Exceptional Children, 19*(3), 12–14.

Jones, C., & Lorman, J. (1991). *Dysarthria: A guide for the patient and family.* OH: Interactive Therapeutics.

Kleppe, S., Katayana K., Shipley, K., & Foushee, D. (1990). The speech and language characteristics of children with Prader-Willi syndrome. *Journal of Speech and Hearing Disorders, 55,* 300–309.

Knoblauch, B. (1998, October). *Teaching children with Tourette syndrome.* ERIC Clearinghouse on Disabilities and Gifted Education (ERIC EC). Available: (online): http://www.cec.sped.org/digests/e570.htm

Kuban, K., & Leviton, A. (1994). Cerebral palsy. *New England Journal of Medicine, 330*(3), 188–195.

Layton, T., & Watson, L. (1995). Enhancing communication in nonverbal children. In K. A. Quill (Ed.). *Teaching children with autism: Strategies to enhance communication and socialization* (pp. 73–103). New York: Delmar.

Leshin, L. (1997–1998). *Trisomy 21: The story of Down syndrome.* Available (online): http://www.ds-health.com/trisomy.htm

Levine, N. (1990). Curing cleft lips and palates. *USA Today, 119,* 4.

MacMillan, D. L. (1982). *Mental retardation in school and society* (2nd ed.). Boston: Little, Brown.

March of Dimes Birth Defects Foundation. (1995, November). *Cleft and lip palate.* White Plains, NY. March of Dimes. NOAH Team. Available (Online): http://www.noah.cuny.edu/pregnancy/march_of_dimes/birth_defects/cleftlip.html

March of Dimes Birth Defects Foundation. (1999). *Oral-facial clefts.* Available (Online):
http://www.modimes.org/HealthLibrary2/FactSheets/Oral_facial_clefts.htm

Mastropieri, M., & Scruggs, T. E. (2000). *The inclusive classroom: Strategies for effective instruction.* Upper Saddle River, NJ: Merrill/Prentice-Hall.

Moran, M., & Pentz, A. (1995, Spring). Helping a child with a cleft palate in your classroom. *TEACHING Exceptional Children, 27*(3), 46–48.

National Down Syndrome Society. (n.d.). *About Down syndrome.* Available (Online): http://www.ndss.org/AboutDS/aboutds.html

National Information Center for Children and Youth with Disabilities. (1991). *General information about Down syndrome.* Fact Sheet no. 4 (FS 4). Washington, DC: Author.

National Information Center for Handicapped Children and Youth with Disabilities. (1995). *Cerebral palsy.* Washington, DC: Author.

National Institute of Neurological Disorders and Stroke. (1996, May). *Cerebral palsy— Hope through research.* National Institutes of Health, Bethesda, MD. Available (Online): http://www.intelihealth.com/IH/ihIH

Peterson, N. L. (1987). *Early intervention for handicapped and at-risk children.* Denver, CO: Love.

Phelps, L., & Grabowski, J. (1992). Fetal alcohol syndrome: Diagnostic features and psychoeducational risk factors. *School Psychology Quarterly, 7*(2), 112–128.

Pinkerton, D. (1991, November). *Substance Exposed Infants and Children.* ERIC Clearinghouse on Disabilities and Gifted Education (ERIC EC). [online]. Available: http://www.cec.sped.org/digests/e505.htm

Prader-Willi Syndrome Association. (1998, May). *Educating the child with Prader-Willi syndrome.* [online]. Available: www.pwsa-uk.demon.co.uk/educatn.htm

Quill, K. A. (1995). *Teaching children with autism: Strategies to enhance communication and socialization.* New York: Delmar.

Ratner, N. (1997). Atypical language development. In J. Gleason (Ed.), *The development of language* (pp. 348–397). Boston: Allyn & Bacon.

Reed, V. A. (1994). *An introduction to children with language disorders* (2nd ed.). New York: Merrill/Macmillan.

Rynders, J. E., & Horrobin, J. M. (1990). Always trainable? Never educable? Updating educational expectations concerning children with Down syndrome. *American Journal on Mental Retardation, 95*(1), 77–83.

Saskatchewan Special Education Unit. (1998). *Teaching students with autism: A Guide for Educators.* [online]. Available: http://www.sasked.gov.sk.ca/curr_inst/speced/educate.htm

Scherer, N. (1999) The speech and language status of toddlers with cleft lip and or palate following early vocabulary intervention. *American Journal of Speech-Language Pathology, 8,* 81–93.

Schubert, A. (1997). "I want to talk like everyone": On the uses of multiple means of communication. *Mental Retardation, 35*(5), 347–354.

Shiminiski-Maher, T. (1989). Selective posterior rhizotomy in the pediatric cerebral palsy population: Implications for nursing practice. *Journal of Neuroscience Nursing, 21*(5), 308–312.

Texas Pediatric Surgical Associates. (n.d.). *Cleft lip and cleft palate.* Available (Online): http://www.pedisurg.com/PtEduc/Cleft_Lip-Palate.htm

Tourette's ruins lives. Orlando Sentinel (1998, December 6), A-25.

Tourette Syndrome Association. (1997). *Tourette syndrome.* Bayside, NY: Author.

Turnbull, A., Turnbull, R., Shank, M., & Leal, D. (1999). *Exceptional lives. Special education in today's schools* (2nd ed.). Upper Saddle River, NJ: Merrill/Prentice-Hall.

Twachtman, D. (1995). Methods to enhance communication in verbal children. In K. A. Quill (Ed.), *Teaching children with autism: Strategies to enhance communication and socialization* (pp. 133–162). New York: Delmar.

United Cerebral Palsy Association. (1993). Facts and figures about cerebral palsy. *Fact Sheet.* Washington, DC: Author.

VanBorsel, J. (1997). Articulation in Down syndrome adolescents and adults. *European Journal of Disorders of Communication, 31,* 415–444.

Vergason, G., & Anderegg, M. L. (1997). *Dictionary of special education and remediation.* Denver, CO: Love.

Wehman, P. (1992). *Life beyond the classroom: Transition strategies of young people with disabilities.* Baltimore: Brookes.

Willard-Holt, C. (1998). Academic and personality characteristics of gifted students with cerebral palsy: A multiple study. *Exceptional Children, 65*(1), 37–50.

11

Augmentative/Alternative Communication and Assistive Technology

Gwendolyn Alexander and Martha S. Lue

Chapter Objectives

On completion of the chapter, the reader will be able to identify and list:

- Legislative mandates that support the use of augmentative/alternative communication systems and assistive technology devices and services for persons with disabilities;
- Characteristics of people who may benefit from the use of assistive technology devices and services;
- Various categories of assistive technology devices and resources; and
- Strategies that the classroom teacher might use with a student with disabilities in an inclusive setting.

- John M. is enrolled in the Varying Exceptionalities program at the local high school. He is new at the school, and little is known about his background. He currently lives with his grandmother, and comes to school on a regular basis. John appears to be functioning at a high level; he is very sociable, and is eager to participate in class discussions and activities. However, his speech is difficult to understand; it consists of a series of grunts, but few true words are understood. When he came to the school, he used the augmentative device *Liberator,* but now refuses to carry it or to use it. The teacher has found a unique software program, *Boardmaker,* which includes functional pictures that he will be able to use as a part of a communication wallet. In the meantime, John continues to make his needs known by merely grunting.

- Eric has cerebral palsy, a condition that severely limits his mobility and ability to communicate. Each day, Eric has many opportunities to interact with his peers and family. However, his expressive language skills are limited. While attending school, Eric developed excellent left-hand motion, which enabled him to use basic sign language and an electric wheelchair. Although these were important achievements, Eric still could not communicate his basic needs and desires to others.

  Initially, a manual communication board (MCB) consisting of the alphabet and numbers was used. When initiating conversation or responding to others, Eric pointed to each letter in the word or phrase to spell out his message. This communication method was a slow and laborious process that was frustrating for both Eric and his communication partners. In spite of all of his communication strategies, Eric ended up nodding either YES or NO to a series of questions, rather than spelling out his messages.

  At the age of fifteen, Eric met a student who used an electronic voice output communication device. At that point in his life, Eric was determined to have a voice of his own. After a thorough assessment of his communication needs, including a trial use of several voice output communication devices, the Touch Talker was selected as the communication system that best met Eric's needs. Finally, Eric could speak to people using his own voice. Assistive technology changed Eric's life, enabling him to become independent and confident in his interactions with his family and friends.

Both *John* and *Eric'*s stories present examples of individuals who benefit from the use of augmentative/alternative communication systems. Augmentative/alternative communication systems have opened the avenue for access to education, employment, and independent travel, as well as leisure time activities for many individuals with cognitive, physical, and communication disabilities. These systems, including assistive technology, may include adapted toys, computers, eating systems, powered mobility, augmentative communication devices, special switches, and thousands of commercially available adapted solutions to improve an individual's ability to learn, compete, work, and interact with family and friends (RESNA Technical Assistance Project, 1992).

At an ever increasing rate, technology is helping overcome what once were viewed as insurmountable physical and psychological barriers to independence for people with disabilities. The first section of this chapter will explore landmark legislative decisions that have made a significant impact on the development and implementation of assistive technology devices and services in the last decade. In the succeeding sections of the chapter, categories of assistive technology, including augmentative communication devices, will be explored. The concluding sections of the chapter focus on candidates for assistive technology, educational considerations, and other relevant teaching resources. Let us begin with a discussion on assistive technology.

Mandates for Assistive Technology

The widespread use of technology by people with disabilities is still a relatively new phenomenon. For example, after World War II, research laboratories began designing artificial limbs for injured soldiers returning home from the war. Eventually clinics emerged that match technology to the needs of rehabilitation patients.

In recent years, the federal government, in lending and supporting use of technology, recognized the significant role that technology may play in the lives of individuals with disabilities. With the passage of the *Technology-Related Assistance for Individuals with Disabilities Act of 1988 (TECH Act), (P.L. 100-407),* in August, 1988, Congress acknowledged the powerful role assistive technology can play in maximizing the independence of individuals with disabilities. This was the first law passed by Congress with the sole purpose of expanding the availability of assistive technology via implementation of consumer-responsive statewide programs for individuals of all ages with disabilities.

The two major components of the Tech Act are: the Title I and Title II programs. The Title I program was established to provide discretionary funds to states on a competitive basis. It also provided technical assistance to states to assist in developing statewide consumer-responsive programs of technology-related assistance for people with disabilities. Title II authorized the funding of assistive technology programs that are of national significance to identify barriers that impede access to assistive technology and/or facilitate access to assistive technology devices and services.

The Education for All Handicapped Children Act (EHA, P.L. 94-142), passed in 1975, and its amendments, on the other hand, mandated a free and appropriate public education (FAPE) for children and youths with disabilities. The EHA makes it possible for states and localities to receive federal funds to assist in the education of infants, toddlers, preschoolers, children, and youths with disabilities. To remain eligible for federal funds under the law, states must ensure that:

- All children and youths with disabilities, regardless of the severity of their disability will receive a free, appropriate public education;
- An Individualized Education Program (IEP) and Individualized Family Service Plan (IFSP) will be drawn up for each child who is eligible for special education–related services or early intervention services;

- To the maximum extent appropriate, all children and youths with disabilities will be educated in the regular education environment;
- Children and youths receiving special education have the right to receive related services necessary to fully benefit from special education instruction;
- Parents have the right to participate in every decision related to the identification, evaluation, and placement of their child;
- Parents must give consent for any initial evaluation, assessment, or placement;
- The right of parents to challenge and appeal any decision related to the identification, evaluation, and placement, or any issue concerning the provision of the EHA, is fully protected and clearly detailed in the due process procedures; and
- Parents have the right to confidentiality of information (RESNA Technical Assistance Project, 1992).

In 1986, the EHA was amended and the eligibility for special education and related services for all children with disabilities was lowered from the age of five to age three, beginning with the 1991–1992 school year. This amendment also established the *Handicapped Infants and Toddlers Program (Part H),* which provides services for infants and toddlers from birth to age two. For infants and toddlers, assistive technology may be specified in the Individualized Family Service Plan (IFSP) and include toys and other devices that develop readiness skills that will enhance the child's participation in both the home and educational environments.

During 1990, the name of the law was changed from the *Education for All Handicapped Children Act* to *the Individuals with Disabilities Education Act (IDEA).* At this time, assistive technology and transition services were added as new amendments to be included when developing a child's IEP.

The definitions of assistive technology devices and services as incorporated in the TECH Act and IDEA are as follows:

> *Assistive Technology Device* means any item, piece of equipment or product system, whether acquired commercially off-the-shelf, modified or customized, to increase, maintain, or improve functional capabilities of individuals with disabilities.
>
> *Assistive Technology Service* is any service that directly assists an individual with a disability in the selection, acquisition, or use of an assistive technology device. This service includes:
>
> - Evaluation of the technology needs of the individual, including a functional evaluation in the individual's customary environment;
> - Purchasing, leasing or otherwise providing for the acquisition of assistive technology devices for individuals with disabilities;
> - Selecting, designing, fitting, customizing, adapting, applying, maintaining, repairing, or replacing of assistive technology devices;
> - Coordinating and using other therapies, interventions, or services with assistive technology devices, such as those associated with existing education and rehabilitation plans and programs;

- Providing assistive technology training and technical assistance with assistive technology for an individual with a disability, or, where appropriate, the family of an individual with disabilities;
- Providing training or technical assistance for professionals, employers, or other individuals who provide services to, employ, or otherwise are substantially involved in the major life functions of individuals with disabilities (RESNA Technical Assistance Project, 1992).

An earlier significant piece of legislation that was passed is Section 504 of the Rehabilitation Act of 1973. Students who have orthopedic impairments, but do not qualify for special education services, may be eligible for special accommodations under this law. This means that schools may need to make special arrangements so these students will have access to a full range of programs and activities.

The Americans with Disabilities Act (ADA) (1990) defines disability as any condition that impairs major life activities such as seeing, hearing, walking, or working. The purpose of this law is to eliminate barriers that exist in five major areas: accessibility and accommodation requirements in public facilities, employment, transportation and communication, state and local government services, and equal opportunity.

One of the rights and protections addressed in the ADA is the requirement that an employer with fifteen or more employees cannot discriminate against a person with a disability who "fits" the job qualifications or who can perform the job with reasonable accommodations. Reasonable accommodation is defined as some modification in a job's task or structure, or in the workplace, that will enable the qualified employee with a disability to do the job. These modifications or changes can include assistive technology and technology access. Modifications must be made, unless they create an undue hardship for the employer.

These legislative decisions made a tremendous impact on incorporating the use of assistive technology in educational programs, employment, and community life. With the implementation of the Tech Act, IDEA, and ADA, states are more responsive to the assistive technology needs of all individuals with disabilities.

ASHA and Assistive Technology

The American Speech-Language-Hearing Association (1991) put forth the following position statement on individuals who are nonspeaking and who may exhibit, to some degree, neurological, emotional, physical, or cognitive disabilities:

> In order to provide effective communication systems for individuals whose speech is not fully functional a number of communication techniques have been developed which are in widespread use . . . nonverbal, alternative, assistive, augmentative, supplementary, aphonic, prosthetic, and aided. (p. 9)

Blackstone (1989) estimated that between 2.5 percent and 6 percent of special needs youngsters are in need of augmentative, alternative communicative services.

Included in this number are youngsters with disabling conditions, such as cerebral palsy, mental retardation, sensorial impairments, and brain and spinal cord injuries.

Reflection

As a group, share your own thoughts on this reflection:

In every state, children and adults with disabilities and professionals are learning about "best practices" in the field of assistive technology service delivery. Increased awareness of what is possible and the delivery of services in a multidisciplinary approach will enable individuals with disabilities to be part of the decision-making team to identify the most appropriate technology to enhance their ability to function. This paves the way for new opportunities for individuals with disabilities and their families to receive appropriate assistive technology services within the community in which they live, learn, and work. It will empower the previously ignored citizen who wanted to contribute and prosper in our society.

Activity

Review the Tech Act, IDEA, and ADA and determine how these laws impact persons with disabilities within your community.

Communication Barriers Encountered by Students

The purpose of this section is to provide the reader with a foundation on which to build his or her own perspective of the purpose that assistive technology devices and services should serve for persons with disabilities. As you review the following two case studies, ask yourself the following questions:

- Is assistive technology beneficial for people with disabilities?
- Was the quality of life of the user enhanced by using assistive devices?
- When using a communication device, was the user able to communicate his or her needs effectively?

Case Study A

Rodney was born with congenital hydrocephalus (excess accumulated cerebrospinal fluid in the cranial cavity, resulting in undue pressure on the brain). A surgical procedure (shunt) is usually required to reduce the pressure. He is nonambulatory and totally dependent on his caregivers for all of his needs. Throughout the day, Rodney has many opportunities to communicate with others. His classroom teacher developed a visual display consisting of realistic pictures of items in the classroom environment. Photographs were also used to represent family members and favorite places within the community. The pictures were attached to a clear plexiglass display with Velcro and mounted to his wheelchair.

To make requests at school and home, Rodney's communications partners stand in front of him, and follow his eye-gaze to the selected picture. To confirm the selection, Rodney's communications partners point to the selected picture and ask him if this is what he wants. At that time, Rodney will either blink his eyes one time to indicate "yes" or two times for "no." Rodney can now make his needs known to others and participate in a variety of activities at school and in other settings. The picture sets may be easily changed to fit special events or activities.

Case Study B

Cindy was born in 1983 with a mixed type of cerebral palsy that affects all of her extremities. Although Cindy has some functional speech, it is not clearly understood unless one is familiar with her daily routine and communicative patterns. At home, Cindy uses her natural speech and augments it with signing. Occasionally, problems occur when unfamiliar people attempt to communicate with her. This is especially true when people unfamiliar with sign language try to interpret her requests.

In 1993, Cindy began to use a portable voice output communication device. This device is mounted onto her wheelchair. For written communication, Cindy uses a computer. This allows her to keep pace with her assignments at school and correspond with relatives living in other areas of the country.

Many changes are taking place in our society that affect people with disabilities. When using assistive devices and/or alternative communication strategies, people with disabilities can participate in a wide array of activities and enhance their overall quality of life.

Candidates for Assistive Technology

Assistive technology is crucial for individuals with disabilities. It serves as a vehicle for participating in educational and religious settings or other daily activities. Also, use of these systems may foster independence in mobility as well as communication in the work environment or leisure time activities.

Candidates for assistive technology may include infants and toddlers who have disabilities and children and adults with a wide range of disabilities ranging from learning disabilities to students with cerebral palsy. For a growing number of individuals, however, their ability to communicate verbally has been impaired because of birth defects, trauma, injury, intellectual capacity, or for many other reasons. Therefore, being unable to communicate and/or having a physical disability can adversely affect all aspects of a person's life.

For many individuals with neuromuscular problems, such as severe cerebral palsy or limited cognitive or physical disabilities, speech alone, even with today's technology, may not be a viable means of communication. The degree to which the speech mechanism is affected may limit the amount and quality of their communication skills. These individuals will need to supplement their minimal intelligible speech with another communication system in order to successfully interact with others.

There is no prerequisite for candidates for assistive technology. Individual needs for assistive technology must be assessed on a case-by-case basis. When considering decisions about assistive technology, a thorough knowledge of the student's abilities, limitations, daily responsibilities, and activities is essential. This can be accomplished through a multidisciplinary team assessment with the student and his or her family included as active team participants.

Reflection

The multidisciplinary team consists of a group of professionals from different disciplines who assess the individual needs of the child. Through communication and collaboration, the multidisciplinary team formulates recommendations on all aspects of the child's problems that fall within their area of expertise. The parents and the child and the teacher are an integral part of the team. In your opinion, who would be some of the other members or professionals on the team?

Parent involvement at this assessment stage is vital, especially for children with language and communicative disorders. The information provided from the parents is particularly valuable to the evaluation team because it is derived directly from the child's language patterns and communicative interactions displayed in a wide array of environmental settings.

Activity

As a group, list several ways assistive technology devices and services can enhance the lives of persons with congenital, degenerative, or acquired disabilities.

Collecting Information from Parents

There are several approaches to collecting information from parents. One approach is to use an interview format. During the interview, parents answer a series of questions regarding their child's communication patterns, and other strategies or communication methods currently utilized at home. Another method of collecting information from parents is to request that they complete a questionnaire including the child's developmental history and language functioning. Both of these approaches of data collection should be used to supplement information derived from direct observation(s) of the child.

When the assessment is complete, the team reconvenes to review the results. At that time, an intervention plan is formulated. If an augmentative and alternative communication (AAC) system is recommended, it is crucial to involve the entire family in the training and use of the device(s). The multidisciplinary team serves as a coach for the family and school personnel directly responsible for daily interactions with the child. Both caregivers and school personnel provide the encouragement, support, and assistance needed for the child to confidently use their system to its fullest.

Finally, whether a child continues to use unaided modes of communication or an AAC system, communication partners should remember the following:

- Children will not acquire language unless they are placed in language-rich environments and are given every opportunity to use it on a daily basis.
- Children need communication partners that will stimulate and respond to their communicative attempts.
- As a result of this type of interaction, children will want to learn and use their acquired language/system.

Activity

There are many other conditions in which assistive technology devices and services may enhance life functions. List five such conditions and explain why these devices and services would be helpful.

Categories of Assistive Technology

Assistive technology is configured into several basic categories. These categories provide a framework for organizing information and describing services, and a basis for a common language on technology applications. Assistive technology devices comprise a wide variety of aids, tools, and equipment used by individuals with disabilities to function more effectively in the classroom, home, and workplace (Glennen & DeCoste, 1997). Moreover, when used properly, assistive devices may help assist students in overcoming a vast array of physical and sensorial problems (Smith, Finn, and Dowdy, 1993).

Some categories of assistive technology aids and devices include:

Aids for daily living: A broad general term applied to self-help aids for use in basic living activities such as eating, bathing, cooking, dressing, toileting, home maintenance;

Communication aids: Refers to both electronic and nonelectronic devices that provide a means for expressive and receptive communication for persons without speech. This includes augmentative communication/speech aids/alarm systems, telephone communication aids, assistive listening devices, and visual/reading aids;

Computer applications: Include, but are not limited to, input and output devices (voice, Braille), alternate access aids (headsticks, light pointers), modified or alternate keyboards, switches, and special software that enable persons with disabilities to use a computer;

Environmental control systems: Primarily electronic systems that enable someone without mobility to control various appliances, electronic aids, security systems, and so on, in their workplace, home, or other surroundings;

Home/worksite modifications: Structural adaptations, fabrications in the home, worksite, or other area (ramps, lifts, bathroom changes) that remove or reduce physical barriers for an individual with a disability;

Prosthetics and orthotics: Include replacements, substitutions or augmentation of missing or malfunctioning body parts with artificial limbs or other orthotic aids (splints, braces, etc.);

Seating and positioning: Refer to accommodations or modifications to a wheelchair or other seating system to provide greater body stability, trunk/head support and an upright posture, and reduction of pressure on the skin surface (cushions, contour seats, lumbar supports, for example);

Sensory aids for persons with hearing or visual impairments: Aids used to augment or replace neurophysical handicaps. These might include magnifiers, Braille, speech output devices, large-print screens, hearing aids, TDDs, and visual alerting systems for specific populations;

Wheelchairs/mobility aids: May be manual and electric wheelchairs, mobile bases for custom chairs, walkers, three-wheel scooters, patient lifts, and other utility vehicles for increasing personal mobility;

Transportation aids: Covers adaptive driving aids, hand controls, wheelchair and other lifts, modified vans or other motor vehicles used for personal transportation.

These assistive technology devices may help students with reading problems that result from sensory deficits or learning disabilities to obtain information that would have otherwise been impossible. For example, children with severe speech impairments may use an augmentative and alternative communication (AAC) device to enhance their unaided modes of communication. AAC devices are self-contained units designed to meet the communication needs of children and adults who are unable to communicate through speech. The availability of this rapidly changing type of technology will increase in the future and therefore make it easier for students who require such devices for optimal learning.

Occasionally, students with physical impairments may require alternative access methods to produce written output or operate household appliances and other environmental control devices. These methods enable people with physical impairments to incorporate this type of technology into their daily routine. Students diagnosed with emotional disabilities may, for example, use computers at home or school, with software designed to strengthen their problem-solving skills and their self-esteem.

Alternative input methods for persons with disabilities are now a standard feature in many places, on the telephone, in theme parks, in airports, and government offices. For example, a touch screen and/or voice recognition system, which allows control of a computer through verbal commands, is frequently used. Perhaps these will soon be a part of all communication in our lives.

In summary, there are many categories of assistive technology devices. Often, within each category are subcategories of specific aids and devices. For example, switches can be classified by their type (sip and puff, lever single, or dual, etc.). A thorough assessment of the child's skills and needs can help determine what category of assistive technology is suitable for his or her lifestyle and career goals.

Activity

After reading this section, observe people in your community and/or workplace and determine what assistive devices they use and for what purpose.

Augmentative and Alternative Communication

Each form of species has a communication system, but none is as elaborate as the human communication system. Verbal communication is the highest form of communication and the most intricate of all human abilities. The human vocal tract, which, like a complex musical instrument, has a number of ways of shaping sounds, creates speech, Kurtweil (1989) notes. For example, the vocal folds vibrate, creating a distinctively pitched sound. The length of tautness of the vocal folds determines the pitch in the same way that the length and tautness of a violin or piano string determines its pitch.

Persons in need of augmentation or supplementation of their communicative system use alternative communication strategies. Included in this number are students with disabling conditions, such as cerebral palsy, brain, and/or spinal cord injuries. The field of AAC continues to evolve and undergo changes. This section seeks to explore goals of an AAC program and some common AAC aids available that enable persons with disabilities to participate in special and regular education programs.

Augmentative communication systems, according to the American Speech-Language-Hearing Association (ASHA), refers to the total functional communication system of an individual, which includes a communication technique, a symbol set or system, and communication/interactive behaviors (ASHA, 1991). The terms, *augmentative* and *alternative communication* (ACC), as defined by Glennen & De-Coste (1997) refer to "aided or unaided communication modes used as a supplement to or as an alternative to oral language, including gestures, sign language, picture symbols, the alphabet, and computers with synthetic speech" (p. 772).

In the AAC community, several issues and concerns are frequently noted among professionals who provide AAC services to persons with disabilities: integrated AAC services, interdisciplinary cooperation, AAC user involvement, and vocabulary selection (Schlosser & Lloyd, 1991).

Blackstone (1989) provides an extensive review of goals related to AAC service delivery and program development: (1) defined missions with clear goals; (2) comprehensive identification and evaluation services; (3) adequate equipment and materials for all; (4) commitment to individual needs; (5) family participation; (6) professional and knowledgeable staff; and (7) efficient and effective administration. The recognition of the need for "best practices" in the area of AAC service delivery warrants further exploration of these goals. For example, a program described by Blackstone seeks to assist persons in three ways:

- Center-based model, wherein persons come to the center for help;
- Community-based model, wherein help comes to the people;
- Collaborative model, which represents a combination of both.

Goals for an AAC program, suggests Blackstone, are to assist individuals with their daily communication needs and to help them facilitate the development of or return of speech and language skills.

Facilitated Communication

In June, 1961, R. C. Oppenheim's story, "They Said Our Child Was Hopeless" appeared in the *Saturday Evening Post*. In this story, the author reports that her six-year-old son, identified as autistic, learned to write his name and some words with minimal support and guidance from her hand. She described a method, later identified as facilitated communication, which at that time was not widely known or utilized.

Facilitated communication is a method used to enhance communication through a facilitator who provides emotional and physical support to the hand, wrist, arm, or shoulder of a person as they use either an electronic communication device or manual system to initiate or respond to messages from their communication partners. As the person with the disability and her or his facilitator become familiar with this method of communication, physical support may be gradually reduced over time. Children and adults with autism, severe cerebral palsy, mental retardation, and other developmental disabilities use this method of communication (Schlosser & Lloyd, 1991; Simpson & Myles, 1995; Zangari, Lloyd, & Vicker, 1994).

The author of facilitated communication, its present name, is Dr. Rosemary Crossley (Crossley & Remington-Guerney, 1992) of Australia. Douglas Biklen (1990) learned of her work, traveled to Australia to observe it, and later wrote about it (Biklen, 1992; Biklen & Schubert, 1991). Since that time, numerous authors have written about this technique. For some users, it has provided increased involvement in academics, social participation, and self-advocacy (Schubert, 1997). As with many new techniques, controversy does exist. For example, do the typed messages represent the thoughts of the facilitator rather than those of the autistic child? Other unanswered questions include:

- Will this technique work for all students with disabilities?
- How does cognitive and language functioning affect the effectiveness of this technique?
- Can more than one facilitator work with the child at any given time?

In one study, researchers suggest that a mechanical device be designed to replace the human facilitator, and thus obviate the charge that the child's hand was manipulated. Berger, Billings, Edelson, and Rimland (1998) evaluated the device, the augmentative hand support system. The system consisted of an easel that held the keyboard, a steel coil spring clamped to the desktop, and a T-bar and arm support attached to the top of the spring. Results of the study indicated that the device did not enable nonspeaking autistic subjects to communicate in writing, nor could the participants communicate via standard facilitated communication.

In summary, until further research and validation of this method is completed, gaining reliable answers to these questions and others will continue to concern both supporters and critics (Jacobson, Mulick, & Schwartz, 1995; Heward, 2000). Substantial validation of the facilitated communication method will provide: (1) information to consumers that will assist them in making the best choice of communication methods, thus meeting the needs and learning styles of their child; (2) guidelines for implementation; (3) school districts and community agencies with information regarding resources, training, and personnel available to support the use of this method. In reference to the area of training, Jacobson, Mulick, and Schwartz remind us that

> practitioners who themselves lack the skills to evaluate the effects of controversial or unproven treatments have an obligation to assure that appropriate evaluation of treatment effect occurs. (p. 762)

Activity

Review three journal articles on facilitated communication. Summarize each article and reflect on the benefits versus the drawbacks of using the facilitated communication approach to enhance communication.

Technological Applications

Use of computers and similar technologies to augment or enhance verbal or written communication appears to be widespread. Computer-based communication devices enable persons with physical disabilities to function more independently within the classroom, community, or work environment. In this section, we will explore computer-based applications and intervention strategies that are used to enhance educational services for students with disabilities.

Writing Systems

There are many writing systems available for students with physical disabilities. These systems are comprised of four basic components (Glennen, 1997):

- Computer base
- Word-processing software
- Adaptive input devices (keyboard, joystick, mouse, etc.)
- Output devices (printers, speech output devices)

In this writing system, the software provides the basic text entry and editing functions, while an adaptive input device provides the method by which all entries are made into the computer. Lastly, the selected output device is used to provide, for example, either speech output or a hard copy of all correspondences through the use of a printer.

Peripherals

Peripherals, such as input and output devices, are of particular interest to teachers and therapists. These devices are most often modified for students with disabilities. Four common input devices are (McCormick & Schiefelbusch, 1990):

- **Light pens used with specialized software.** As the user directs the light onto the monitor, the light controls the image, allowing the user to either draw or write on the screen. For students who have good head control and limited mobility in their hands, attach the light pen to either a headband or eyeglasses for use.
- **Touch-sensitive pads and graphics tablets.** These devices can attach to the computer and serve as drawing tablets. Students may use an isolated finger or another adaptive aid as an input device.
- **Touch screens.** Touch screens are used as an alternative to a keyboard. Students simply touch the screen to respond. Touch screens are attached directly to the computer's monitor with a Velcro strip. The monitor itself may be touch sensitive.
- **Alternative keyboards.** These input devices either replace or supplement the standard keyboard.

There is a wide range of software programs available for use with children to familiarize them with the computer. These programs are designed to teach alphabet recognition and math concepts, and reinforce cause-and-effect relationships. Some programs require the use of a single switch, power pad, touch screen, or Echo speech synthesizer.

Assistive Technology and Students with Visual Impairments

Students with visual impairments have the same basic needs as most students. This developmental process begins at birth. With the first touch, kiss, or other act of affection, the visually impaired child begins to develop a sense of trust and security. With continuous parental nurturing and support, visually impaired infants or children will learn that they too can achieve their highest educational potential.

In spite of the latest technological advancements in the medical arena, there are many children born with visual impairments that may limit their functional capabilities. Some children will be diagnosed as visually impaired at a later period in their life. Still others will have either a structural or pathological condition of the eye that may be identified at birth. Using their residual vision, these children most likely will be able to function adequately throughout their lives. Another group of children will have medical conditions that will progressively worsen later in life. Sooner or later, these degenerative conditions often result in a loss of visual functioning sometime during the child's school years. Occasionally, accidents or disease result in a loss of visual functioning and/or blindness among children.

There are a growing number of children with visual impairments that have no intelligible speech. These children may also have other disabilities that limit their functional ability. For these children, more than one visual problem can occur. This may result in many hours of assessment and equipment trials to determine the most appropriate AAC system to meet their needs. It is important for the evaluation team to take into consideration the following factors of vision that affect the selection and use of an AAC system: visual acuity, visual fields, oculomotor functioning, light sensitivity, cortical vision, and color sensitivity.

There are many useful assistive devices for children with visual, physical, and resulting communication impairments. This wide range of devices will help the child receive information and learn, as well as communicate with others. Some of these systems include devices that scan, convert, and print documents into speech and portable devices that convert print images into tactile configurations via raised vibrating pins. Others include talking books and magazines, small portable Braille note-takers, closed-circuit TVs, magnifying systems, alternate keyboards, hardware and software enhancements for computers, and optical character recognizers. Just the miniaturization of electronics is making devices more available and efficient.

For children with visual impairments, assistive devices can serve as a catalyst to help them master a variety of tasks, enhance their opportunities for socialization, and participate in a wide array of educational experiences. At this time, we are just beginning to understand the impact assistive devices can have on the development of children with visual impairments. With continuous progress in this area, we can enhance educational opportunities, work and community environments, and employment options, for both children and adults with visual impairments.

Reflection

Record your reflections to this statement:
- Assistive technology continues to improve and provide more opportunities for persons with disabilities. It is imperative that we continue to strive to find new ways to promote use of this equipment within our communities.

Positioning and the Use of Augmentative and Alternative Communication Systems

The introduction of an augmentative communication system is often a frustrating experience for children, therapists, families, or teachers. Without proper positioning, their best efforts may fail, and an expensive piece of equipment will be abandoned. Therefore, successful use of a communication aid or technique can be directly attributed to proper seating. For example, positioning of students with cerebral palsy can have a major impact on their abilities to function effectively, including the ability to communicate. The position, if possible, that usually provides the greatest benefit is the upright, seated position in a wheelchair or other chair (McEwen & Lloyd, 1990).

Developing a cooperative relationship between the physical and occupational therapist, speech-language pathologist, teacher, and parent is vital to the success of the AAC program. Each team member's goals may be different. For the physical therapist, for example, positioning goals may include:

- Achieving stability, support, and proper alignment, decreasing the likelihood of contracture and skeletal deformities;
- Normalizing muscle tone to decrease the influence of abnormal reflexes and facilitate normal movements;
- Making the client comfortable, thus providing a sense of safety and minimizing fatigue.

Keep in mind however, that other members of the team (e.g., a speech-language pathologist) may present additional requirements and seating goals. These goals may include:

- Improving breathing to enhance speech;
- Facilitating swallowing and decreasing drooling;
- Improving arm and hand function, making it easier to use an augmentative communication aid and/or gestures or sign.

Abnormal reflexes, diminished respiration, and bodily discomfort all interfere with cognitive activities. The following list contains seating and positioning needs of the augmentative communication user:

- Upright posture and best possible head control;
- Adequate respiration to support speech;
- Minimizing fatigue and increasing session length;
- Improved hand function to operate augmentative devices;
- Alternative body site for operating adaptive switches.

In summary, before beginning any assessment procedures or implementation of AAC aids and/or activities, it is essential that the student be appropriately positioned to achieve optimal visual, upper extremity, and motor performance.

Activity

Review three journal articles on the use of positioning techniques for persons with disabilities that use adaptive devices. Summarize each article and reflect on the benefits derived from proper positioning and use of assistive devices.

Funding Options

The issue of providing funding for assistive technology devices and services is not new. For many years, caregivers, school personnel, occupational and physical therapists, speech clinicians, and other professionals who provide services for students with disabilities have searched for possible funding sources for assistive technology devices (Parette, Jr., Hoffman, & VanBiervliet, 1994).

Several possible funding sources currently exist for assistive technology devices and services: Medicaid, private insurance companies, vocational rehabilitation programs, trust funds, private corporations, public/private fund-raisers, nonprofit civic organizations, and school districts (DePape, 1988). Keep in mind that the application process varies from organization to organization.

Before applying for an assistive technology device, it is imperative that the child have a comprehensive assessment, including an equipment trial period, to determine the most appropriate device to meet his or her needs. At this early stage, it is important for the child and the family to get hands-on experience in using a device prior to purchase.

When a decision is reached as to the type of device or service needed, the next step is to identify the funding source. If, for example, Medicaid or private insurance is being considered, the parents must follow the steps outlined by that particular agency for securing an assistive technology device or service.

The *key* to funding any device is justification. If the parents or evaluation team are requested to write a justification letter, it should focus on the need for the device and the potential to help the child interact with family and peers, participate in the educational setting, and prepare her or him to meet future goals in the workplace. Above all, this letter of justification must include relevant information that supports the claim that this device and/or service will enhance the child's overall independent functioning. Information provided in the justification letter should include:

- Background information, including a medical diagnosis, skills and abilities, and communication limitations;
- Description of the evaluation process, including equipment trials;
- Description of the recommended device and its cost, including repair and maintenance;
- Letter of medical necessity or prescription.

Many funding sources require that a letter of medical necessity be included in the funding application packet. This letter can be obtained either from a physician, speech pathologist, or other medical professional who works directly with the child. Progress reports or additional evaluations should also be submitted to further support the case.

In some letters of medical necessity, a communication device is referred to as a *communication prosthesis*. This aid serves to support the child's educational, medical, and vocational needs. When including this information in the letter of medical necessity, it is important to state why this particular prosthetic device will meet the individual needs of children, for example:

- Convey basic needs and wants, so children can be less dependent on their parents for interpretation of messages and care;
- Gain the attention of others when help is needed;
- Participate in discussions and decisions that involve them and their immediate family; and
- Convey information about medical history to a physician.

Most insurance companies and state and federal programs have an appeals process. Before requesting an appeal, explore the procedure. Many companies will request additional information to substantiate the claim, while others may request a hearing before a claims officer. In the latter case, the client, family, and funding advocate will have an opportunity to present their case that could include a demonstration of the equipment being considered.

In summary, funding for assistive technology devices and services may be a long process. Careful documentation from professionals who work with the child, medical information obtained from a physician, and the results of a comprehensive assessment, including equipment trials, will justify the need for this equipment to the funding source.

Activity

Draft your own letter of medical necessity for one of the vignettes presented in the chapter.

What a Teacher Needs to Know about Assistive Technology

In some early intervention programs or classrooms for students with disabilities, teachers are confronted with the continuous challenge of teaching without a set curriculum. This may result in students obtaining "splinter" skills throughout their educational experiences. If a specific curriculum is followed, however, there may be little emphasis placed on incorporating the use of assistive technology within the classroom setting (Fuller, Lloyd, & Schlosser, 1992; Glennen, 1997).

Incorporating the use of a curriculum will provide a foundation for the teacher and a framework for activities and skills students should master at various developmental stages. This curriculum will also serve as an accountability measure for school districts throughout the nation as we strive to meet increased educational standards.

A challenge arises when children with disabilities are included in regular education programs. Many classroom teachers have never been introduced to a specific curriculum for students with disabilities nor have they experienced having them in their classroom. To facilitate a smooth transition into a regular classroom, the special education teacher or assistive technology coordinator, if available, should collaborate on the use of technology in the classroom, being sensitive to the strengths and weaknesses of the student, classroom environment/arrangement, and daily schedules and routines. The classroom teacher should make a conscious effort to attend any training, meetings, or other activities where the needs and learning style of the student with disabilities are discussed.

Once the teacher is familiar with the student and his or her goals, the student can then be slowly mainstreamed into the regular education class. Classmates and other school personnel should learn about the child's modes of communication, including the use of specific assistive technology devices. All students should be encouraged to interact with students with disabilities and communicate with them using their communication system. The teacher may wish to incorporate a variety of games into the daily routine such as "Simon Says," "Go Fish," or a guessing game. These games are highly motivating, can have multiple players, and will encourage communication interactions. As children engage in these activities with their nondisabled peers, they will begin to feel part of the classroom community.

The teacher may also want to solicit assistance from the community or school volunteers to assist in the classroom. These volunteers can provide many hours of assistance with small groups and one-on-one instruction. In some schools, volunteers serve as mentors, provide technical assistance for computers and other technologies, operate technology loan libraries, and provide support for families of students with disabilities.

In summary, teachers should be aware that the curriculum is just as important for a student with a disability as it is for regular education students. As more students with disabilities are mainstreamed in regular education classrooms, teachers should be aware of the specific needs and assistive technology devices that enhance their educational and vocational programs for special needs students. Furthermore, assistive technology may be incorporated at varying stages of the child's life; each teacher should remember that the technology utilized is vital to the child's transition from school to college or a vocational setting. For more in-depth discussion of assistive and augmentative communication, readers are refered to Blackstone (1989), Beukelman & Mirenda (1992), and Glennen & DeCoste (1997).

Reflection

Share your reflections regarding the following statements:
- **Outstanding teachers continuously look for ways to enhance instruction, especially teachers confronted with the challenge of mainstreaming students with disabilities into regular education programs. For this task to be successful, cooperation and collaboration is needed between the family of the child with disabilities, the child, therapists, and school officials.**
- **Communication with all of the families of all students in a class is particularly crucial. The teacher needs not only their support, but their understanding of the challenges ahead. The parents should be assured that their child will continue to be challenged academically and that the child with disabilities will not detract from instruction or eliminate opportunities for other students to advance academically.**

Activities

- Interview teachers who have students with disabilities mainstreamed into their regular education classrooms. List four things the teachers had to accomplish in order to prepare their classroom for these students. You may want to include additional materials needed, courses/workshops attended that assisted the teacher for the student with disabilities, and support received from the staff/administration during this process.
- Adapt four games that are commercially available to use with a student with disabilities. Explain how the adaptation will help the student involved.
- Review three journal articles on strategies teachers can use when mainstreaming students with disabilities into regular education programs.

Summary

Writing this chapter on assistive technology has enabled the authors to see the continued need for improvement in the area of service delivery for students with disabilities. Although we have made significant strides in our methodology, we are a long way from providing complete assistance for all persons with disabilities.

The various case studies cited help us to appreciate the benefits derived from using assistive technology devices to enhance the functional abilities of students with disabilities. These students can share their thoughts, feelings, and actions, participate in reading activities within their classroom setting, and maintain contact with important persons in their environment such as a doctor or teacher. They can also express personal needs such as the desire to use the bathroom or inform their caregivers of an illness or injury.

Teachers, caregivers, and other professionals who provide services for students with limited communication skills should remember that alternate communication strategies are best utilized in natural environments in the context of purposeful activities. These children will learn to communicate through parent–child or teacher–child interactions in real conversations, when making real requests for assistance, and when answering and asking questions that relate to a specific subject. Whether a child uses an assistive device or a manual communication system to accomplish these tasks, communication partners should be informed, patient, and supportive during this process.

In conclusion, assistive technology plays a vital role in enhancing the lives of persons with disabilities. It is imperative that we continue to explore ways to enhance these services and improve the quality of assistive devices for future users and our own knowledge of needs assessment for the devices and the use of devices when available.

Vendors, Journals, and Resource Centers

It is the assumption of the authors that teachers, especially beginning teachers, could benefit from a listing of vendors, resource centers, and commonly used terms associated within the area of assistive technology.

The following list contains various assistive technology devices and services that may be either purchased or utilized by teachers, parents, and school districts. This listing is provided to familiarize the reader with the many companies that manufacture assistive technology products today. These resources are listed together for easy retrieval and study.

As the area of assistive technology continues to change, so will its products. They will become more sophisticated, economical, and valued by society in general. Professionals and caregivers will need to keep abreast of current information and changes in this area so that they, too, can make informed decisions regarding the use of assistive technology devices and services within their community.

Vendors

Adaptive Aids
P.O. Box 13178
Tucson, AZ 85732

Adaptive Communication
Systems, Inc.
354 Hookstown Grade Road
Clinton, PA 15026

Crestwood Company
P.O. Box 04606
Milwaukee, WI 53204

Developmental Equipment
P.O. Box 639
Wauconda, IL 60084

Dragon Systems, Inc.
55 Chapel Street
Newton, MA 02158

Imaginart
30 Arizona Street
Bisbee, AZ 85603

Steven Kanor
8 Main Street
Hastings-on-Hudson, NY 10706

Mayer-Johnson Company
P.O. Box 1579
Solana Beach, CA 92075-1579

Prentke Romich Company
1022 Heyl Road
Wooster, OH 44691

Telesensory Systems, Inc.
P.O. Box 7455
Mountain View, CA 94039-7455

ADAM Lab
Wayne County Intermediate Schools
33500 Van Born Rd.
Wayne, MI 48184

Communication Skill Builders
3130 North Dodge Boulevard
P.O. Box 42050
Tucson, AZ 85733

CompuAbility Corporation
101 Route 46 East
Pine Brook, NJ 07058

Don Johnson Developmental Equipment
200 Winnetka Terrace
Lake Zurich, IL 60047

Edmark Corporation
14350 North East 21st St.
Bellevue, WA 98009-3903

Innocomp
33195 Wagon Wheel
Solon, OH 44139

Kurzwell Applied Intelligence, Inc.
411 Waverly Oaks Road
Waltham, MA 02154-8465

Phonic Ear Inc.
250 Camino Alto
Mill Valley, CA 94941

Sunburst Communications
39 Washington Avenue, Room EP
Pleasantville, NY 10570

TASH (Technical Aids & Systems
   for the Handicapped)
70 Gibson Drive, Unit 12
Markham, Ontario, Canada L3R 4C2

Unicorn Engineering Co.
6201 Harwood Avenue
Oakland, CA 94618

Words +, Inc.
P.O. Box 1229
Lancaster, CA 93535

VTEK, Inc.
1625 Olympic Boulevard
Santa Monica, CA 90404

Zygo Industries, Inc.
P.O. Box 1008
Portland, OR 97207

Journals

AAC Augmentative and Alternative Communication
[journal]
P.O. Box 785
Lewiston, NY 14092-0785

Augmentative Communication News [newsletter]
Sunset Enterprises
One Surf Way, Suite 237
Monterey, CA 93940

Augmentative Speaking Newsletter
912 Niblick Dr.
Casselberry, FL 32707

Closing the Gap [newspaper]
Rt. 2, Box 39
Henderson, MN 56044

Communicating Together
Easter Seal Communication Institute
P.O. Box 986
Thornhill, Ontario Canada L3T 4A5

Communication Outlook [newsletter]
Artificial Language Laboratory
Michigan State University
405 Computer Center
East Lansing, MI 48824-1042

Journal of the Association for Persons with Severe Handicaps
11201 Greenwood Avenue, North
Seattle, WA

Journal of Visual Impairments and Blindness
The Sheraton Press
450 Paine Avenue
Hanover, PA 17331

Journal of Special Education Technology
Peabody College, Box 328
Vanderbilt University
Nashville, TN 37203

Exceptional Children and *Teaching Exceptional Children*
The Council for Exceptional Children (CEC)
1920 Association Drive
Reston, VA 20191-1589

Resource Centers

The Adriana Foundation
2001 Beacon Street, Suite 214
Brookline, MA 02146

American Foundation for the Blind
National Technology Center
15 W. 16th Street
New York, NY 10011

American Speech-Language-Hearing Association
(ASHA)
10801 Rockville Pike
Rockville, MD 20852

The Association for Persons with Severe Handicaps
(TASH)
7010 Roosevelt Way NE
Seattle, WA 98115

The Council for Exceptional Children (CEC)
and
ERIC Clearinghouse on Disabilities and Gifted Education
1920 Association Drive
Reston, VA 22091-1589

Foundation for Technology Access
2173 E. Francisco Blvd., Ste. L
San Rafael, CA 94901

International Society for Augmentative and Alternative Communication (ISSAC)
P.O. Box 1762
Station R
Toronto, Ontario, Canada M4G 4A3

National Federation of the Blind
1800 Johnson Street
Baltimore, MD 21230

Sensory Access Foundation
399 Sherman Avenue, Ste. 12
Palo Alto, CA 94306

National Information Center for Children and Youth with Disabilities (NICHCY)
P.O. Box 1492
Washington, DC 20013-1492

March of Dimes Birth Defects Foundation
P.O. Box 1657
Wilkes-Barre, PA 18703

References and Suggested Readings

American Speech-Language-Hearing Association. (1991). Report: Augmentative and alternative communication. *ASHA, 33 (Suppl. 5)*, 9–12.

American Speech-Language-Hearing Association. (1993). Definitions: Communication disorders and variations. *ASHA, 35 (Suppl. 10)*, 40–41.

Americans with Disabilities Act. (1990). P.L. 101-336.

Bebko, J. M., Perry, A., & Bryson, S. (1996). Multiple method validation study of facilitated communication II. Individual differences and subgroup results. *Journal of Autism & Development Disorders, 26*, 19–42.

Berger, C. L., Billings, D., Edelson, S. M., & Rimland, B. (1998). Evaluation of a mechanical hand-support for facilitated communication. *Journal of Autism & Development Disorders, 28*, 153–157.

Beukelman, D. R., & Mirenda, P. (1992). *Augmentative and alternative communication: Management of severe communication disorders in children and adults*. Baltimore, MD: Paul H. Brookes.

Biklen, D. (1990). Communication unbound: Autism and praxis. *Harvard Educational Review, 60*, 291–314.

Biklen, D. (1992). Typing to talk: Facilitated communication. *American Journal of Speech-Language Pathology, 1*, 15–17.

Biklen, D., & Schubert, A. (1991). New words: The communication of students with autism. *Remedial and Special Education, 12*, 46–57.

Blackstone, S. (1989). Augmentative communication services in the schools. *ASHA, 3*, 61–64.

Bomba, C., O'Donnell, L., Markowitz, C., & Holmes, D. L. (1996). Evaluating the impact of facilitated communication on the communicative competence of fourteen subjects with autism.

Journal of Autism & Developmental Disorders, 26, 43–58.

Crossley, R., & Remington-Guerney, J. (1992). Getting the words out: Facilitated communication training. *Topics in Language Disorders, 12*, 29–45.

DePape, D. (1988). Guidelines for seeking funding for communication aids. Trace Research and Development Center, 6–7.

Dollars and Sense, A Guide to Solving the Funding Puzzle and Getting Assistive Technology in Georgia. Georgia Department of Human Resources, Division of Rehabilitation Services, Tools for Life.

Education Act for All Handicapped Children Act. (1975). P.L. 94-142.

Fuller, D. R., Lloyd, L. L., & Schlosser, R. W. (1992). Further development of an augmentative and alternative communication symbol taxonomy. *Augmentative and Alternative Communication, 8*, 67–74.

Glennen, S. L. (1997). Augmentative communication systems. In S. L. Glennen & C. DeCoste (Eds.), *Handbook of augmentative communication* (pp. 59–96). San Diego: Singular Publishing Group.

Glennen, S. L., & DeCoste, C. (1997). *Handbook of augmentative communication*. San Diego: Singular Publishing Group.

Handicapped Infants and Toddlers Act. (1986). P.L. 99-457.

Heward, W. L. (2000). *Exceptional children* (6th ed.). Upper Saddle River, NJ: Merrill/Prentice-Hall.

Jacobson, J. W., Mulick, J. A., & Schwartz, A. A. (1995, September). A history of facilitated communication: Science, pseudoscience, and anti science. *American Psychologist, 50,* 750–765.

Kurtweil, R. (1989). Beyond pattern recognition. *BYTE,* 277–288.

McCormick, L. P., & Schiefelbusch, R. L. (1990). *Early language interventions: An introduction* (2nd ed., pp. 305–306). Boston: Allyn & Bacon.

McEwen, I. R., & Lloyd, L. L. (1990). Positioning students with cerebral palsy to use augmentative and alternative communication. *Language, Speech, and Hearing in the Schools, 21,* 15–21.

Oppenheim, R. C. (1961, June 17). "They said our child was hopeless." *Saturday Evening Post, 234,* 23, 56–58.

Parette, Jr., H. P., Hoffman, A., & VanBiervliet, A. (1994, Spring). The professional's role in obtaining funding for assistive technology for infants and toddlers with disabilities. *TEACHING Exceptional Children, 26,* 22–28.

Parette, Jr., H. P., Hourcade, J. J., & VanBiervliet, A. (1993, Spring). Selection of appropriate technology for children with disabilities. *TEACHING Exceptional Children, 25,* 18–22.

Public Law 100-407 (1988). Technology Related Assistance for Individuals with Disabilities Act. Section 3.

RESNA Rehabilitation Engineering & Assistive Technology Society at North America Technical Assistance Project. (1992). *Assistive Technology and the Individualized Education Program* (pp. 1–5, August). [online]. Available: http://www.resna.org

Schlosser, R. W., & Lloyd L. (1991). Augmentative and alternative communication: An evolving field. *Augmentative and Alternative Communication, 7,* 154–160.

Schubert, A. (1997). "I want to talk like everyone." On the use of multiple meanings of communication. *Mental Retardation, 35,* 347–354.

Simpson, R. L., & Myles, B. S. (1995). Effectiveness of facilitated communication with children and youth with autism. *Journal of Special Education, 28,* 424–439.

Smith, T. E. C., Finn, M. D., & Dowdy, C. A. (1993). *Teaching students with mild disabilities.* Orlando, FL: Harcourt Brace Jovanovich.

Technology-Related Assistance for Individuals with Disabilities Act. (1988). P.L. 100-407.

Technology-Related Assistance for Individuals with Disabilities Act Amendments. (1994). P.L. 103-218.

Zangari, C., Lloyd, L. L., & Vicker, B. (1994). Augmentative and alternative communication: An historic perspective. *Augmentative and Alternative Communication, 10,* 27–59.

Collaboration: The Role of the Speech-Language Pathologist and the Special Educator in the Inclusive Process

Martha S. Lue

Chapter Objectives

On completion of this chapter, the reader will be able to:

- Compare and contrast the professions of speech-language pathology and special education;
- Identify several models of delivery of services for individuals with disabilities; and
- Describe the role of some of the members of the team serving children with disabilities.

- Meredith is enrolled in the communicative disorders undergraduate program at the university. During her final semester, she decided to take a course in exceptional education. She chose the general survey course in exceptional education. For the first time in her undergraduate career, she interacted with preservice educators outside her major discipline. In her reflective journal, she recorded the following:

  > I've learned so many different aspects of special education. What's more important is that I'm able to develop strategies that may be used in the classroom.

The amount of work and research, lecture, and hands-on experiences, as well as visiting classes with children with special needs have all led to a better understanding of the profession and the importance of the collaborative process in meeting the needs of all of our children.

- Each weekday morning, the Family Support Team meets at the local school to discuss students who may be in need of additional services. Members of the team include a speech-language pathologist, guidance counselor, classroom teacher, social worker, and school psychologist. Today they are discussing Louis, a nine-year-old child from Haiti. His teacher was concerned because he wasn't remembering what he heard, his academics were extremely low, he did not know sounds and sight words, and, overall, had made no progress in reading. He spoke Haitian-Creole and was being seen in the bilingual program. The team recommended hearing and speech referral to the speech-language pathologist; the classroom teacher was going to employ the use of a peer buddy; the social worker was going to make a home visit to communicate with the parents. Louis was going to receive individual tutoring twenty minutes a day, four days a week. The classroom teacher will keep the team abreast of his progress.

- Patricia serves as a school psychologist on a diagnostic team in her local school district. The team consists of a speech-language pathologist, the audiologist, and an assistive technology specialist. This week, they are discussing Joseph, a five-year-old. A visit with Joseph's mother indicated that he was "acting out a lot, using profanity, and taking things." The mother was not always able to understand his speech, describing it as if "he is dragging his tongue." After evaluations from the team of specialists, he was diagnosed as developmentally delayed with behavioral problems.

Meredith will someday be a very important member of a collaborative team. The *Family Support Team* and the *school psychologist* cases indicate the need for increased dialogue among all professionals involved with working with children in inclusive settings. As mandated under the Individuals with Disabilities Education Act (IDEA) and Section 504 of the Rehabilitation Act of 1973, schools are required to provide a variety of services for students with disabilities. These services may range from transportation, health, and medical or psychological counseling to those provided by speech-language pathologists (Dettmer, Dyck, & Thurston, 1999). Further, PL 94-142, the Education for All Handicapped Children's Act (EHA), a forerunner of The Individuals with Disabilities Act (IDEA), mandates the use of multidisciplinary teams to determine student eligibility for special education and appropriate placement, and to monitor the individual's progress after placement. The 1999 reauthorization of IDEA (PL 105-17) included general provisions that encourage the placement of students with disabilities in inclusive settings. For this to take place, a process for identifying the needs or problems and for exploring modifications that address them must be used. One such model is called *collaboration.*

This chapter will explore the dynamics of collaboration. The history of special education and speech-language pathology will be examined. Models for delivery of services for professionals will be addressed. Finally, the supporting role of members of the team serving children with disabilities will be addressed.

In traditional school settings, children's academic and social–emotional needs are usually met through the individual efforts of general and special educators (Coben & Thomas, 1997). But a 1996 report from the U.S. Department of Education indicated that nearly three fourths of students with disabilities receive their instructional programs in regular education and resource room settings; 95 percent of students with disabilities are served in regular education schools (Salend & Duhaney, 1999). As we move toward meeting the needs of students with disabilities in inclusive settings, different professionals with different roles are needed to meet the specific needs of students with disabilities. One of the keys to successful integration for individuals with disabilities is *collaboration,* for these students will require various combinations of services during their school years. For the special educator, this is not new. Smith and Luckasson (1995) explain that special educators collaborate in many ways: with parents and families, in performing multidisciplinary assessments, in developing individualized family service plans (IFSPs) and individualized education plans (IEPs), and in the development of individualized transition plans (ITPs) from school to work.

Reeve and Hallahan (1994) describe collaboration in this manner:

> During initial implementation of 94-142, school systems focused on establishing self-contained programs for students with disabilities, a service delivery model popular in the 1960s . . . [In] the 1970s and early 1980s, this emphasis changed with the resource model of delivery service. . . . Recently, the calls for educational reform, special education restructuring, and full inclusion have provided further impetus for collaboration between general and special educators. (p. 1)

Speech-Language Pathology: The Profession

A speech-language pathologist is a specialist in the study of speech and language and in the treatment of speech-language disorders. An audiologist is a specialist in the study of hearing, hearing disorders, and in the assessment and rehabilitation of hearing impairments (Hedge, 1995). While they work in a variety of settings, as outlined in Figure 12.1, many still work in public school settings (ASHA, 1995). For the school-based speech-language pathologist, the role continues to evolve (Harn, Bradshaw, & Ogletree, 1999). As a member of the collaborative team, the speech-language pathologist has the primary responsibility for identifying, assessing, and providing therapeutic services for those individuals with communication problems (Lowe & Angelo, 1993; Hunt & Marshall, 1999). These duties may also include (Hunt & Marshall, 1999):

- determining what may have caused the onset & development of the problem;
- determining whether other factors contribute to the maintenance of the problem; and
- clarifying the problem for both the student and family, counseling them appropriately.

As noted by Paden (1970), the first speech and hearing programs in the public schools began in Chicago in 1910, where it was observed that problems in speech and hearing affected children's performances in the classroom (Boone & Plante, 1993). Speech and hearing services were made available in the schools

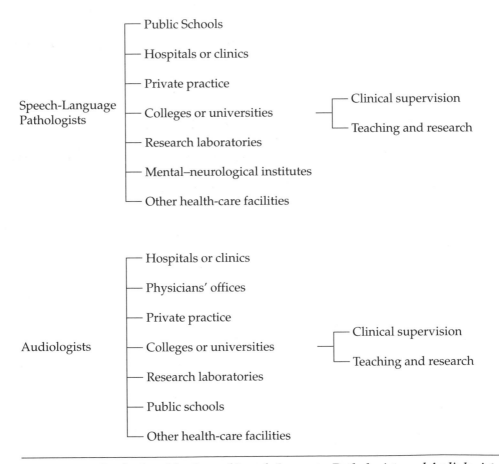

FIGURE 12.1 *Professional Settings of Speech-Language Pathologists and Audiologists*

From Hedge, M. N. (1995). Specialists in communication and its disorders. In *Introduction to communication disorders* (2nd ed., p. 59), Austin, TX: PRO-ED.

rather than sending the children to a clinic or hospital, thereby necessitating the possible loss of valuable instructional time. Figure 12.2 highlights that history (Paden, 1970; Matthews & Fratalli, 1994; Bloodstein, 1984). Over the years, both the

FIGURE 12.2 *Field of Speech-Language Pathology: A Historical Perspective*

Early 1900s	University of Iowa created an academic discipline by combining several departments in the university and selecting an outstanding student.
1910	Ten speech correctionists hired in Chicago public schools
1910	Two speech correctionists employed in Detroit public schools
1913	Speech training program begun in New York City for children who had speech impairments
1913	Boston schools began a program of speech correction
1916	Programs established in the New York and San Francisco areas
1916	Eight cities in the state of Wisconsin had speech correction teachers
1918	Publication of paper, "How to begin speech correction in the public schools." Author: Walter B. Swift
1915	First speech clinic established at a university, University of Wisconsin
1921	First Ph.D. granted in the field of communication disorders; awarded to Sarah M. Stinchfield
1924	Lee Edward Travis granted a Ph.D., later became director of program at University of Iowa.
1925	American Academy of Speech Correction organization established
1935	Changed name to American Speech Correction Association
1947	Name of association changed to American Speech and Hearing Association
1978	Organization's name changed to American Speech-Language-Hearing Association, but maintained its original abbreviation, ASHA.

services and the organization that we know as the American Speech-Language-Hearing Association (ASHA) have continued to grow (Bender, 1982).

The American Speech-Language-Hearing Association

The American Speech-Language-Hearing-Association (ASHA) is the professional and scientific association for more than 96,000 speech-language pathologists, audiologists, and speech, language, and hearing scientists in the United States and internationally. The mission of the ASHA is to promote the interests of and provide the highest quality services for professionals in audiology, speech-language pathology, and speech and hearing sciences, and to advocate for people with communication disabilities (American Speech-Language-Hearing Association, 1998).

From ancient times speech difficulties in individuals have interested people, yet speech pathology is a young discipline that emerged only in the 1920s. In 1925, a small number of leading scholars in the field formed a group called the American Society for the Study of Disorders of Speech. As the professional organization grew, it took on the name American Speech and Hearing Association. Speech and hearing clinicians began to gain prominence and could be found in hospitals, rehabilitation centers, schools, and universities. In 1978, the association changed its name to American Speech-Language-Hearing Association. Speech and language disorders are becoming a global concern and the profession is growing via publications, professional organizations, and collaboration with related professions.

Since 1936, ASHA has published scientific and technical journals for the speech and hearing field: *Journal of Speech and Hearing Disorders* and *Journal of Speech and Hearing Research*. Its website address is *http://www.asha.org*

ASHA's Code of Ethics

Lowe (1993) observed that acceptable standards of professional and ethical behavior of their members are defined by all professional organizations that make up the human service delivery system. For this purpose, a code of ethics is usually established. For the speech-language pathologist and audiologist, the American Speech-Language-Hearing Association's code of ethics is used. Silverman (1999) observed that ethical issues have been of paramount concern since the Association's founding in 1925. While, during the early years, the concerns were primarily those of preventing unethical practitioners from joining, the current code of ethics deals with situations that the speech-language pathologist or audiologist might encounter.

> The preservation of the highest standards and integrity and ethical principles is vital to the responsible discharge of obligations in the professions of speech-language pathology and audiology. Rules of ethics are specific statements of minimally acceptable professional conduct or prohibitions. There are four domains that specific principles of ethics are written for:

- Individuals shall honor their responsibility to the welfare of the persons they serve;
- Individuals shall honor their responsibility to achieve and maintain the highest level of professional competence;
- Individuals shall honor their responsibility to the public by promoting understanding of the profession, supporting the development of services designed to fulfill the unmet needs of the public, and by providing accurate information in all communications involving any aspect of the profession;
- Individuals shall honor their responsibility to the professions and their relationships with colleagues, students, and members of allied professions. (ASHA, 1992) (ASHA, 1998) [online]. Available: http://www.asha.org./ library/code_of_ethics.htm

Special Eduation: The Profession from a Historical Perspective

The field of special education has undergone many changes throughout its history. Many disciplines have contributed to the emergence of the profession—medicine, psychology, sociology, and general education have all been involved in the development of the field.

In the 1900s, attempts at educating students with disabilities in the United States included segregated education or total exclusion from public education entirely. Between 1920 to 1960, programs for students in public schools for disabilities were sporadic and selective. For children with severe emotional problems, mental hospitals were used. Special education programs were allowed, not mandated (Hardman, Drew, & Egan, 1999).

The 1950s brought about an increase in the number of public school classes for students who had been diagnosed as mentally retarded and those with behavior disorders. In 1954, in the groundbreaking case of *Brown v. Board of Education* of Topeka, Kansas, the U.S. Supreme Court established the right of all children to an equal opportunity for an education. The ruling reversed the "separate but equal" doctrine and established the principle that social segregation denies the constitutional rights associated with equality of education.

In the 1960s, Dr. Lloyd Dunn, in his seminal article, "Special education for the mildly retarded—Is it too much or is it justifiable?" opined that too many children were inappropriately being placed in special education programs that were designed to work exclusively with individuals who were mentally retarded. Many of the youngsters in the program were those coming from minority and/or poverty backgrounds. Also in the 1960s, the idea of integrating individuals with disabilities into the larger society was becoming an increasingly popular trend that has continued over the years. Beginning in the 1960s and 1970s, parents and advocates of students with disabilities began to use courts in an attempt to force states to provide an equal educational opportunity for these students (Yell, Rogers, & Rogers, 1998).

Deinstitutionalization was a movement that occurred in the 1960s that involved removing individuals from institutions and integrating them into society. Two landmark cases that involved the concept of equal opportunity for students with disabilities were the *Pennsylvania Association for Retarded Citizens (PARC) v. Commonwealth of Pennsylvania* and *Mills v. Board of Education of Washington, D.C.* (1972). In the Pennsylvania case, the court held that the state of Pennsylvania could not exclude special education children from the public schools and that children with mental retardation were entitled to homebound tutoring and similar services.

In *Mills v. Board of Education of Washington, D.C.* (1972), seven children had been excluded from the Washington, D.C. public schools because of learning and behavior problems. The D.C. Board of Education reported that there was not enough money to provide special education for them. The U.S. Supreme Court ruled that the Board of Education of the District of Columbia had to provide an education for the plaintiffs and any other children similarly situated by accepting and then providing a comprehensive plan of services for children with physical and mental handicaps between the ages of three and twenty-one. Further, it was the duty of the district to hire special education teachers to comply with the court order (Zepada & Langenbach, 1999). The court also ruled that financial problems could not be allowed to have a greater impact on students with disabilities than on students without disabilities (Heward, 1996). The impact of Mills reinforced legislation passed by 45 state legislatures during the 1960s and 1970s, mandating, encouraging, and/or funding special education programs (Center for the Future of Children, 1996).

The Education for All Handicapped Children's Act (EHA) was passed in 1975. The Act, amended in 1990, to be called the *Individuals with Disabilities Education Act* (IDEA), and reauthorized in 1997, addressed issues governing eligibility for special education services, parental rights, individualized education programs (IEPs), the rights of children to be served in the least restrictive environment (LRE), and the need to provide related (noneducational) services. Children with disabilities between the ages of three and twenty-one, regardless of the type and severity of their disability, shall receive a free, appropriate public education without cost to the child's parents. Further, the law changed the language used to identify an individual with a disability to "person first" and also replaced the term *handicapped* with *individuals with disabilities.*

Since the passage of IDEA, 90 percent fewer children with developmental disabilities are living in institutions. Hundreds of thousands attend public schools and regular classrooms. Three times as many are enrolled in colleges and universities. Twice as many individuals in their twenties are in the U.S. workplace (Yell, Rogers, & Rogers, 1998). These improvements in the well-being and quality of life for individuals with disabilities are the result of almost a century of parents, advocates, and individuals with disabilities themselves fighting to achieve the equality and rights that they deserve.

Another important movement that was passed by federal legislation took place in the 1980s, the regular education initiative (REI). This legislation required general education teachers to take greater responsibility for students with special needs.

Two influential organizations, the Council for Exceptional Children (CEC) and the Association for Retarded Citizens (ARC), were pivotal in elevating the issue of special education to a national level (Zepada & Langenbach, 1999).

Council for Exceptional Children: The Profession

The major professional organization in special education is the Council for Exceptional Children. The organization has several specialized divisions that provide information on a specific exceptionality or interest area in special education. Included are divisions for persons interested in learning disabilities, technology and media, teacher education, communication disorders, intellectual deficits, and culturally and linguistically diverse population learners. There are a website address, professional conferences, journals, and opportunities for professional development, monographs, and networking opportunities. The Council for Exceptional Children (CEC) promulgates a *Code of Ethics and Professional Conduct* for teachers and related personnel in special education. The Code ascribes principles for educators and holds them responsible for upholding these principles. Sections of the CEC Code that have special relevance to this discussion are as follows:

- Commitment to quality of life potential of exceptional individuals;
- Promotion of high level of competence and integrity in our profession;
- Engagement of beneficial professional activities for all concerned;
- Exercising of objective professional judgement;
- Working within the standards of the profession.
  (*Code of ethics and standards for professional practice.* Council for Exceptional Children, 1983)

For the special educator, each state determines the criteria that persons must meet for certification in each of the exceptionalities (Swan & Sirvis, 1992). The Council for Exceptional Children has published suggested standards for the initial preparation and certification of teachers of students with disabilities (1994). CEC's website address is *http://www.cec.sped.org*

Collaboration Defined

Members of a collaborative team are viewed as stakeholders (Smalley, Lue, Dziuban, Dumbacher, & Seaton, 1999; McClure, 1998), for the stakeholders are both empowered and enabled by this process. McClure (1998) goes on to state: "They are empowered through the fact that decisions are made collaboratively and they are enabled because the decisions being made are more likely to support what they are trying to accomplish . . ." (p. 2).

The word *collaboration* comes from Latin *collaboratus,* meaning, "to labor to-gether." It can be further defined from a number of different perspectives. It may be viewed as "a style for direct interaction between at least two co-equal parties voluntarily engaged in shared decision making as they work toward a common goal" (Cook & Friend, 1991).

Pfeifer (1980) defines *collaboration* as an organized group of professionals from different disciplines having unique skills and the common goal of cooperative problem-solving. Perhaps Idol, Paolucci-Whitcomb, and Nevin (1986) offered the most comprehensive definition of *collaboration:*

> Collaboration is an interactive process that enables people with diverse expertise to generate creative solutions to mutually defined problems. The outcome is enhanced, altered, and produces solutions that are different from those that the individual team members would produce independently. The major outcome of collaboration is to provide effective programs for students with needs within the most appropri-ate context, thereby enabling them to achieve maximum constructive interaction with their nonhandicapped peers. (p. 1)

Parameters of Collaboration: Opportunities

Collaboration is a growing trend in schools across the nation. Much has been writ-ten about the opportunities and challenges of collaboration. Opportunities include the following:

- There should be mutual goals that are specific enough so that they can be both operationalized and evaluated;
- Individuals should voluntarily participate in the activities (whereby profes-sionals choose to carry out collaborative activities);
- Each must have equally valued personal or professional resources to con-tribute; and
- Individuals involved must be willing to share resources, decision-making au-thority, and accountability for the outcomes of their activity (sharing/assists in the development of a sense of ownership).

Other assets, as outlined by Van Dyke, Stallings, and Colley (1995) include honest and open communication, flexibility, and recognition of differing needs, IEP responsibility, and a sense of humor.

Parameters of Collaboration: Challenges

Inherent in any change process are challenges that must be addressed. The collab-orative model has its own:

- having administrative support;
- making time available for consultation and collaboration (Alpert & Tracht-man, 1980);

- resolving conflicts arising between what educators would like to do and what they are able to do (Evans, 1980);
- improving participation in team meetings (Ysseldyke, Algozzine, & Allen, 1982);
- time limitations, lack of training for team members, and confusion regarding role responsibilities (Tindal, Shinn, & Rodden-Nord, 1990; Kaiser & Woodman, 1985).

Dohan and Schulz (1998) add that collaboration is "planning, implementing, and refining methods of service delivery to meet students' changing requirements in an ongoing process that demands dedication, creativity, and a willingness to acquire new skills" (p. 16).

> *Activity*
>
> **Spend the day with a collaborative team at a local school. What were some of the advantages and disadvantages that you saw in this approach?**

Service Delivery Models for Speech-Language Pathologists and Special Educators

Several educational service options are available for students with disabilities. Traditionally, these options have varied, from including students with disabilities being served in general education classrooms with no additional or specialized assistance, through the option of students being educated through hospital or homebound instructional programs. As mandated by IDEA, students with disabilities must receive their education to the maximum extent appropriate with their nondisabled peers. Schools must, then, develop a continuum of placements, ranging from general classrooms with support services to homebound and hospital programs (Hardman, Drew, & Egan, 1999).

Collaboration can take place in many forms ranging from the more traditional pullout services (Achilles, Yates, & Freese, 1991) to classroom-based speech and language programs (Dohan & Schulz, 1998). The strengths and weaknesses of these models have received attention in the literature (Klinger, Vaughn, Schuman, Cohen, & Forgan, 1998; Galentine & Prelock, 1995; Elksnin, 1997). Harn, Bradshaw, and Ogletree (1999) suggest that collaborative service delivery models are replacing traditional "pull out" approaches in many schools. "The role is also changing in response to myriad developments, both within and outside of communication disorders, and with this changing role, have come new challenges" (p. 163).

Emerging Models

Borsch and Oaks (1993) have described four service delivery models successfully used in collaboration between speech-language pathologists and special educators:

team teaching: In this model, both the classroom teacher and the speech-language pathologist teach in the classroom, teach skills and content, and share the responsibility for planning the lesson, teaching the lesson, monitoring progress of students, and making decisions about modifications needed;

complementary teaching: In this model, it is the classroom teacher who teaches most of the lesson. The speech-language pathologist focuses on related speech and language skills. These colleagues teach in the classroom from their own areas of expertise. As with team teaching, each shares responsibility for planning and teaching the lessons, monitoring the progress, and decision-making about adaptations and modifications;

supportive teaching: This approach, which can occur either in a pull-out setting or in the classroom, involves the speech-language pathologist teaching supplemental information or related to the curriculum while at the same time incorporating speech and language skills in the lesson; and

resource management: Here the speech-language pathologist works outside of the classroom, but goes into the classroom to observe. Both the speech-language pathologist and the teacher plan, monitor, and make decisions about materials collectively.

Reflection

Identify some of the persons involved in the collaborative process. What does each contribute to the team?

Positive Outcomes

When collaboration is presented at its best, everyone—including the classroom teacher, the speech-language pathologists, the students with communication disorders, and all of the other students in the classroom—can benefit. Collaboration has further benefits that Borsch & Oaks (1993) describe:

- Each person learns from the other;
- Each person's skills complement the other's;
- Commitment between professionals increases;
- Responsibility is shared;
- Problem-solving is shared;
- Service delivery is more flexible;
- Inclusion and how it can work are addressed.

Models for Delivery of Services in Special Education

Special education means that specifically designed instruction will be provided that meets the unusual needs of an exceptional learner. This includes the use of special material, teaching techniques, or equipment and/or facilities that may be required (Hallahan & Kauffman, 1997). Students with special needs are educated in a variety of settings: a self-contained approach, wherein the special teacher provides most or all of the instruction in a special class of students; a resource room, wherein the children are pulled out of a regular setting for a given academic or behavioral skill taught by a trained special educator; the regular teacher provides most of the instruction.

Emerging Models

In the past two decades, two models for the delivery of services for students with disabilities have emerged (Coben & Thomas, 1997): consultation and collaboration. Much research has been presented to support both. The consultation model has been traced to the Vermont Consulting Teacher program where highly trained special education teachers served as consulting teachers to assist general education teachers to work with students with disabilities (Cook & Friend, 1991).

The consultation model, as viewed by Tharp (1975), involves three individuals: the consultant, the mediator, and the target. The mediator is described as the professional attempting to bring about a change in the targeted individual; the consultant is one with the expertise regarding strategies to change the behavior.

Activity

View the websites of the American Speech-Language-Hearing Association (ASHA) and the Council for Exceptional Children (CEC). Compare and contrast the mission statements and the code of ethics of each organization. Briefly report on your findings.

The Role of Parents in the Collaborative Process

Working closely with parents is critical. Next to the child, parents are viewed as some of the most important persons in the collaborative process. The relationship should be meaningful and respectful. They should be seen as equal partners. They are much needed and valued members of the team. They are able to provide information related to the child's adaptive behavior, and medical, social, and psychological history (Salend, 1998). Stanovich (1996) adds that

> the most important way to get parents to be seen, and to see themselves, as equal partners is to get them to school . . . attendance at open houses . . . encouraging

parents to serve as volunteers in the classroom . . . drop in whenever they have the chance so that they can observe or help out as needed. (p. 41)

Van Dyke, Stallings, and Colley (1995) observed that if parents were kept abreast of what is taking place in the classroom, they would be supportive of the teacher's efforts. Further, the authors add, "when the classroom community is extended to include parents, greater involvement will lead to greater success" (p. 478). Effective strategies for increased parental involvement might include scheduling meetings at a time that parents can attend and ensuring that information in conveyed in a language that parents could understand (Rainforth & England, 1997).

Collaboration and Collegiality

Collaborative planning and collegial relations have been identified as important variables that are present in effective schools (Purkey & Smith, 1985). It has been reported that these relationships tend to make complex tasks more manageable, may lead to the stimulation of new ideas, and may present opportunities for collaborative teachers to attempt innovations that would exhaust the energy, skill, or resources of one individual teacher (Inger, 1993). In order for this to take place, all persons need to feel valued, comfortable, and respected (Galentine & Prelock, 1995). Further, to insure that this takes place, Rainforth & England (1997) recommend that every team member assume the roles of a learner, a teacher, and implementer. Still another critical aspect of a successful team is the ability to engage in active listening. Strategies for this to take place, as outlined by Gable & Manning (1999), include:

- clarifying the role of each participant;
- organizing one's thoughts before expressing them;
- observing body language (nonverbal cues) of team members;
- avoiding professional jargon; and
- giving credit for the contributions of team members.

In true collaboration, de Fur (1997) notes, "the outcome is something that could not have been achieved by one person or entity alone" (p. 77).

Important Readings on Collaboration

Ogletree (1999) presented an overview of several articles featured in the January 1999 issue of *Intervention in School and Clinic*. The articles are based on five interrelated disciplines on instruction and behavior management. Other issues mentioned include the importance of socially valid practices for the modern special educator and reshaping professional roles for school counselors, psychologists, and speech-language pathologists.

Evans (1991) took a critical look at the research that has been conducted on collaboration in special education. Until recently, much of the information gathered on this topic has come from professionals in fields other than special education. This article strives to examine the literature on collaboration and its relationship to special education. Evans also points out the many flaws in prior research. These flaws include small sample sizes and descriptive rather than quantitative research.

Coben and Thomas (1997) described the consultation, collaboration, and teaming models used among special educators. The authors highlight each model's strengths and weaknesses, as well as the ways in which the models can contribute to interactive teaming. Guidelines for successful implementation of the models are also provided. The authors conclude the article by stressing that collaboration and collegial relationships are vital components of effective schools.

Reeve and Hallahan (1994) addressed the expected roles of teachers, pre-referral intervention through collaborative consultation, elements of cooperative teaching, and the barriers to effective collaboration. In the field of special education, collaboration among general and special educators has become a topic of much attention. Despite the overwhelming amount of attention collaboration has attracted, many questions regarding its effectiveness still exist.

Cooperative teaching, another type of collaboration, is also addressed in the article. This coteaching model has become increasingly popular in recent years and is an excellent way to accommodate inclusive classrooms.

Cook and Friend (1991) define *collaboration* and *consultation*, movements in special education that emerged in the 1990s. The terms encompass many definitions including team meetings, relationships with peers, and working with the parents. Cook and Friend examine the evolution of the trends of collaboration and consultation as used in special education. Consultation takes place when highly trained special education teachers serve as consultants to regular education classroom teachers. Collaboration is a direct interaction between at least two coequal professionals in the schools voluntarily using their resources and knowledge to work toward a common goal.

Dettmer, Dyck, and Thurston (1999) define another model of collaboration, collaboration school consultation as interaction in which school personnel and families confer, consult, and collaborate as a team to identify learning and behavioral needs, and to plan, implement, evaluate, and revise as needed the educational programs for serving those needs. The need for collaboration will continue to grow as our student population increasingly becomes more diverse.

Researchers at the University of Kansas, The Beach Center on Families and Disability, found school inclusion without collaboration to be virtually impossible. Special education students often receive services from many professionals in the school system and coordinated services are needed. A collaborative team can include: speech-language pathologist, physical therapist, school psychologist, program consultants, interpreters, special and general education teachers, occupational therapist, administrators, the student's family, and others. All members of the team should feel they are treated equally and all ideas should be considered.

Harn, Bradshaw, & Ogletree (1999) examined the changing role of speech pathologists. Collaborative services and pull-out programs are changing the role of the speech-language pathologist in our school systems from the traditional role in the 1950s and 1960s. The chief contributor to this need for role change is an increasingly diverse student population in U.S. schools. Inclusion brings on more curriculum-based assessment, and alternate service delivery models require a great breadth of knowledge, all leading to expanded scope of service speech-language pathologist must provide. A detailed case example is provided in the article.

Summary

Today professionals are called on to work with an increasingly diverse population of exceptional learners. This call further presents the opportunity to work with other individuals who will assist in the education of students with disabilities. As we move toward meeting the needs of all students in more inclusive settings, it becomes clear that no single individual has the expertise or resources needed to work with all children. This chapter has addressed the changing roles of the speech-language pathologist and the special educator in the delivery of services to students with disabilities. Traditional service models were described as well as emerging models. The histories of special education and speech-language pathology were highlighted. In this history, three disciplines usually functioned for the most part in isolation and in separate classrooms. But as we continue to provide services for students with disabilities in inclusive settings, collaboration will remain an important and critical factor in school reform. In order for this to be effective, each discipline must be prepared for changing and evolving roles. As with any new and evolving process, time for reflections, to step back and assess "next steps" will need to take place. As described by Galentine and Prelock (1995), sometimes there may be a need for still another individual, a mediator, to assist team members to objectively confront and reconcile differences. "But," they add, "whatever it takes, collaboration is something to strive for, something that will benefit not only the team members but, more importantly, the population being served" (p. 51). Lastly, this process takes patience, perseverance, time, and an awareness of the difficulties inherent in change (Wood, 1998). It will require intentionality and commitment (Rainforth & England, 1997). New patterns of behavior must take place between disciplines, agencies, and all involved (de Fur, 1997).

References and Suggested Readings

Achilles, J., Yates, R., & Freese, J. (1991). Perspectives from the field: Collaborative consultation in the speech & language program of the Dallas Independent School District. *Language, Speech, and Hearing Services in Schools, 22,* 154–155.

Alpert, J., & Trachtman, G. (1980). School psychological consultation in the eighties: Relevance for the delivery of social services. *School Psychology Review, 9,* 234–238.

American Speech-Language-Hearing Association. (1992). Code of ethics, *ASHA, 34*(3) (Suppl. 90), 1–2.

American Speech-Language-Hearing Association. (1995). ASHA 1994 annual report. *ASHA, 37,* 18–26.

American Speech-Language-Hearing Association. (1998). About ASHA [On-line]. Available: http://www.asha.org/professionals/association/about_asha.htm

Beach Center on Families and Disability. (1998, October 26). How to professionally collaborate for effective special education. [online]. Available: http://cmc.mcg.edu.edu/fam_resources/beach_center.htm.

Bender, M. (1982). Roots and wings. ASHA's membership—1925 to 1989. *ASHA, 31,* 76.

Bloodstein, O. (1984). Speech pathology and speech disorders. In O. Bloodstein (Ed.), *Speech pathology: An introduction* (2nd ed., pp. 1–5). Boston: Houghton Mifflin Company.

Boone, D. R., & Plante, E. (1993). *Human communication and its disorders* (2nd ed.). Boston: Allyn & Bacon.

Borsch, J., & Oaks, R. (1993). *The collaboration companion: Strategies and activities in and out of the classroom.* East Moline, IL: LinguiSystems.

Brown vs. Board of Education of Topeka, 347 U.S. 483 (1954).

Center for the Future of Children/The David and Lucille Packard Foundation. (1996, Spring). *Special education for students with disabilities, 6*(1). [online]. Available: http://www.futureofchildren.org/sped/exsum.htm

Coben, S., & Thomas, C. (1997). Meeting the challenge of consultation and collaboration: Developing interactive teams. *Journal of Learning Disabilities, 30,* 427–432.

Cook, L., & Friend, M. (1991). Collaboration in special education. *Preventing School Failure, 35*(2), 4–24.

Council for Exceptional Children. (1983). Code of ethics and standards for professional practice. *Exceptional Children, 50,* 205.

Council for Exceptional Children. (1994, Spring). *CEC standards for professional practice in special education.* Reston, VA: Author.

Council for Exceptional Children. (1998). *What every special educator must know: The international standards for the preparation and licensure of special educators* (3rd ed.) Reston, VA: Author.

de Fur, S. (1997). Collaboration as a prevention tool for youth with disabilities. *Preventing School Failure, 41*(4), 173–179.

Dettmer, P., Dyck, N., & Thurston, L. (1999). *Consultation, collaboration, and teamwork for students with special needs* (3rd ed.). Boston: Allyn & Bacon.

Dohan, M., & Schulz, H. (1998). The speech-language pathologist's changing role: Collaboration within the classroom. *Journal of Children's Communication Development, 20,* 9–18.

Dunn, L. (1968). Special education for the mildly retarded—Is it too much or is it justifiable? *Exceptional Children, 35,* 5 22.

Education for All Handicapped Children's Act of 1975 (EHA). Pub. L. No. 94-1142. 8a stat 773

Elksnin, L. (1997). Collaborative speech and language services for students with learning disabilities. *Journal of Learning Disabilities, 30,* 414–426.

Evans, S. (1980). The consultant role of the resource teacher. *Exceptional Children, 46,* 402–404.

Evans, S. (1991). A realistic look at the research base for collaboration in special education. *Preventing School Failure, 35*(4), 10–13.

Ferguson, M. (1992). Implementing collaborative consultation: The transition to collaborative teaching. *Language, Speech, and Hearing Services in Schools, 23,* 361–362.

Friend, M., & Cook, L. (1996). Collaboration as a predictor for success in school reform. *Journal of Educational and Psychological Consultation, 1,* 69–86.

Gable, R., & Manning, M. (1999, Jan/Feb). Interdisciplinary teaming: Solution to instructing heterogeneous groups of students. *Clearing House, 72,* 182–186.

Galantine, J., & Prelock, P. (1995). Collaborative teaming in supervision: The first year. *Journal of Childhood Communication Disorders, 16,* 49–55.

Gerber, A. (1987). Collaboration between speech-language pathologists and educators: A continuing education process. *Journal of Childhood Communication Disorders, 11,* 107–123.

Hallahan, D., & Kauffman, J. (1997). *Exceptional learners: Introduction to special education.* Boston: Allyn & Bacon.

Hardman, M., Drew, C., & Egan, W. (1999). *Human exceptionality: Society, school, and family* (6th ed.). Boston: Allyn & Bacon.

Harn, W., Bradshaw, M., & Ogletree, B. (1999). The speech-language pathologist in the schools: Changing roles. *Intervention in School & Clinic, 34,* 7.

Hedge, M. (1995). *Introduction to communication disorders* (2nd ed.). Austin, TX: PRO-ED.

Heward, W. (1996). *Exceptional children: An introduction to special children* (5th ed.). Englewood Cliffs, NJ: Merrill/Prentice-Hall.

Hunt, N., & Marshall, K. (1999). *Exceptional children and youth* (2nd ed.). Boston: Houghton Mifflin.

Idol, L., Paolucci-Whitcomb, P., & Nevin, A. (1986). *Collaborative consultation.* Austin, TX: PRO-ED.

Individuals with Disabilities Education Act December of 1990, 20 U.S.C. § 1401 *et Seq.* (1997).

Inger, M. (1993). Teacher collaboration in secondary schools. *Center Focus, 2,* 1–8: [online]. Available:

http://ncrve.berkeley.edu/CenterFocus/ CF2.html

Kaiser, S., & Woodman, R. (1985). Multidisciplinary teams and group decision-making techniques: Possible solutions to decision-making problems. *School Psychology Review, 14,* 457–470.

Klinger, J., Vaughan, S., Schuman, J., Cohen, P., & Forgan, J. (1998, March/April). Inclusion or pullout: Which do students prefer? *Journal of Learning Disabilities, 32,* 148–158.

Lowe, R. J. (1993). *Speech-language pathology and related professions in the schools.* Boston: Allyn & Bacon

Lowe, R., & Angelo, D. (1993). The school-based speech-language pathologist. In R. Lowe (Ed.), *Speech-language pathology for related professions in the schools* (pp. 21–46). Boston: Allyn & Bacon.

Matthews, J., & Fratalli, C. (1994). The professions of speech-language pathology and audiology. In G. Shames, E. Wiig, & W. Secord (Eds.), *Human communication disorders: An introduction* (4th ed., pp. 22–33). New York: Merrill/ Macmillan.

McClure, G. (1998). Shared decision making: The benefits and the pitfalls. {On-line}. Available: http://www.rockyview.ab.ca/bpeak/ mcclure/shared.html/

Ogletree, B. (1999). Practical solutions to the challenges of changing professional roles: Introduction to the special issue. *Intervention in School and Clinic, 34,* 131.

Paden, E. (1970). *A history of the American Speech and Hearing Association, 1925–1958.* Rockville, MD: American Speech-Language-Hearing Association.

Pfeifer, S. (1980). The school-based interprofessional team: Recurring problems and some possible solutions. *Journal of School Psychology, 18,* 388–394.

Purkey, C., & Smith, M. S. (1985). School reform: The district policy implications of the effective schools literature. *The Elementary School Journal, 85,* 352–89.

Rainforth, B., & England, J. (1997). Collaborations for inclusion. *Education and Treatment of Children, 20,* 85–104.

Reeve, P., & Hallahan, D. (1994). Practical questions about collaboration between general and special educators. *Focus on Exceptional Children, 26,* 1–10.

Salend, S. (1998). *Effective mainstreaming: Creating inclusive classrooms* (3rd ed.). Upper Saddle River, NJ: Merrill.

Salend, S., & Duhaney, L. (1999, March/April). The impact of inclusion on students with and without disabilities and their educators. *Remedial and Special Education, 20,* 114–126.

Silverman, F. (1999). *Professional issues in speech-language pathology and audiology.* Boston: Allyn & Bacon.

Smalley, S., Lue, M., Dziuban, C., Dumbacher, T., & Seaton, G. (1999). The use of shared decision-making to bring about reform in an at-risk community. Unpublished manuscript.

Smith, D., & Luckasson, R. (1995). IFSP, IEP, ITP: Planning and delivering services. In *Introduction to special education: Teaching in an age of challenge* (pp. 79–130). Boston: Allyn & Bacon.

Stanovich, P. (1996). Collaboration—The key to successful instruction in today's inclusive schools. *Intervention in School and Clinic, 32,* 39–43.

Swan, W., & Sirvis, B. (1992). The CEC common core of knowledge and skills essential for all beginning special education teachers. *Teaching Exceptional Children, 15,* 16–20.

Tharp, R., (1975). The triadic model of consultation, In C. Parker (Ed)., *Psychological consultation in the schools: Helping teachers meet special needs students* (pp. 131–151). Reston, VA: Council for Exceptional Children.

Tindal, G., Shinn, M., & Rodden-Nord, K. (1990). Contextually based school consultation: Influential variables. *Exceptional Children, 56,* 324–336.

Van Dyke, R., Stallings, M., & Colley, K. (1995). How to build an inclusive school community. *Phi Delta Kappan, 76,* 475–484.

Wood, M. (1998). Whose job is it anyway? Educational roles in inclusion. *Exceptional Children, 64,* 181–195.

Yell, M., Rogers, D., & Rogers, E. (1998). The legal history of special education. *Remedial and Special Education, 19,* 219–228.

Ysseldyke, J., Algozzine, B., & Allen, D. (1982). Participation of regular education teachers in special education team decision making. *Exceptional Children, 48,* 365–366.

Zepada, S., & Langenbach, M. (1999). *Special programs in regular schools.* Boston: Allyn & Bacon.

Glossary

AAC: Augmentative/alternative communication.

Abduction: The act of opening the vocal folds.

Adaptation Effect: The increase of fluency caused by successive reading or speaking of the same passage.

Adduction: The act of closing the vocal folds.

Adventitiously Deaf: Loss of hearing after birth, often due to injury or disease.

Affricate: A combination of a stop and fricative ([tʃ], [dʒ]).

Aided: A physical object or device used to transmit or receive messages (e.g., communication book, board, chart, mechanical or electronic device, or computer).

Alveolar: Any consonant made with the tongue near or touching the alveolar ridge: [t], [d], [n], [s], [z].

Alveolar Process: The outer edge of the maxillary bone.

American Sign Language: A visual–gestural language used by deaf or hearing-impaired persons in the United States.

American Speech-Language-Hearing Association (AHSA): Professional organization made up of speech, language, and hearing professionals.

Ankylosis: Restricted use of a bone joint due to disease or restriction of the arytenoids, due to arthritis or cancer.

Anterior: Front.

Apert's Syndrome: Congenital condition characterized by a peaked head and webbed fingers.

Aphasia: Language disorder caused by brain damage due to either stroke or trauma.

Aphonia: Complete absence of voice; loss of voice.

Articulate: In speech, moving the speech mechanism to produce speech sounds.

Articulation: Physiological movements involved in modifying the air flow in the vocal tract above the larynx to produce the various speech sounds; using the structures of the mouth to produce the sounds of speech.

Articulation Disorder: The abnormal production of speech sounds.

Arytenoid Cartilages: Paired pyramid-shaped cartilages attached to each of the vocal folds.

Ataxia: Cerebral damage that causes difficulty with coordination and balance.

Athetoid: Characterized by constant uncontrolled movements, the second most prevalent type of cerebral palsy.

Audiogram: A graph of an individual's hearing level at various sound frequencies.

Audiologist: A nonmedical hearing specialist who tests for hearing sensitivity and administers hearing tests to children and adults with suspected and/or various hearing disorders; a professional trained in audiology.

Audiology: The science dealing with hearing impairments, their detection, and remediation.

Audiometer: Instrument designed to measure the sensitivity of hearing.

Auditory/Vestibular Nerve: Cranial nerve number VIII; its function is sensory control of hearing and balance.

Augmentative Communication: A system used to supplement the communicative skills of individuals for whom speech is temporarily or permanently inadequate to meet communicative needs. Both prosthetic devices and/or nonprosthetic techniques may be designed for individual use for communication.

Autism: A developmental disorder with severe distortions of social and language development that begin at an early age.

Awareness: The teacher's knowledge of the student's specific and individual needs, both within that classroom and those addressed within the IEP.

Babbling: A stage of early language development characterized by the repetition of sounds.

Behavioral Theory: A language theory that focuses on the observable and measurable aspects of language behavior.

Benign: "Kind" tumor; nonmalignant.

Bilabial: Sound made with both lips (/p/, /b/, /m/).

Bilateral Paralysis: Paralysis of both of the vocal folds.

Blade: The tip of the tongue.

Blissymbols: Representational system using pictographs, that depict the outline of the concept presented or ideographs that show the shape of the concept represented. Charles Bliss developed this language system.

Bound Morpheme: One that cannot stand alone, such as a prefix or a word ending.

Brain Stem: Area between the spinal cord and brain hemispheres.

Brown v. Board of Education of Topeka Kansas: A Supreme Court ruling delivered in 1954 that prohibited the use of "separate but equal" schools for African American and Caucasian students.

Carcinoma: Cancer or a malignancy.

Caudal: Tail.

Cephalad: Head.

Cerebellum: Back of the brain stem.

Cerebral Palsy: A neurological condition resulting from damage to the brain before or during birth, or in infancy; it is characterized by disabilities in posture and movement.

Cerebrum: Largest part of the brain.

Class-Wide Peer Tutoring: Strategy wherein all students in a particular class are divided into pairs. Students then assist each other by providing direct instruction and alternate roles of tutor and tutee to master basic academic skills.

Cleft Lip and Palate: Congenital fissure or absence of tissue of the lip and/or palate, premaxilla, and/or velum.

Cluttering: A disorder of fluency often characterized by rapid speech, breaks in fluency, and faulty articulation.

CNS: Central Nervous System; the brain and spinal cord.

Cochlea: The snail-shaped auditory portion of the inner ear.

Cognate: Related sounds ([p][b][t][d][s][z]).

Cognition: The ability to gain knowledge through personal experiences.

Cognitive/Interactionist Theory: This theory points out the relationship between cognition and language, emphasizing the role of experience and the environment in the development of language and focusing on a developmental perspective as a child matures and moves through stages.

Collaboration: A process whereby professionals, including parents, work together with a shared purpose in a mutually beneficial, supportive relationship.

Communication: Written or spoken transmission and reception of information; has at least three components: sender, receiver, message.

Communication Wallet: Communication systems where symbols are categorized by subject and then placed in clear vinyl sleeves. When communicating, the user simply opens the wallet and points to the desired symbol/picture to indicate his or her message.

Communicative Difference/Dialect: A variation of a symbol system used by a group of individuals that reflects and is determined by shared regional, social, and/or cultural/ethnic factors. Variations or alterations in use of a symbol system should not be considered a disorder of speech or language.

Components: All the aids, techniques, symbols, and strategies that are used to supplement or augment the speech of individuals.

Conductive Hearing Loss: Impairment of hearing due to the failure of sound pressure waves to reach the cochlea through the normal air-conduction channels (outer or middle ear).

Congenital: Present at birth.

Congenitally Deaf: Born without hearing.

Consonant: Any speech sound made by constricting the vocal tract enough to impede air flow through the mouth.

Content: A component of language that encompasses meaning or semantics.

Controlling Function: A function of language that is used when the speaker is seeking to influence and control the listener's behavior; persuading and commanding are controlling functions.

Cooperative Learning: An instructional arrangement in which small groups or teams of students work together to achieve a team and individual success in a way that promotes student responsibility.

Coprolalia: Involuntary use of vulgar or obscene gestures or language.

Council for Exceptional Children (CEC): Professional organization made up primarily of educators who work on improving outcomes for individuals with exceptionalities.

Cricoid Cartilage: A ring-shaped cartilage that forms the foundation or base of the larynx.

Curriculum-Based Assessment: Any approach that uses direct observation and recording of a student's performance in the school curriculum as a basis for obtaining information to make further instructional decisions.

Dactylology: finger spelling; also used to include signs as well.

Deaf/Deaf Child: A child whose hearing loss exceeds 90 dB, precluding the understanding of speech through audition.

Decibel (dB): Unit of intensity of sound (loud and soft).

Diphthong: Phoneme produced by the blending of two vowel sounds into a single speech sound.

Distal: Toward the periphery.

Dorsal: Back.

Dorsum: The major part of the tongue.

Down Syndrome: Congenital condition caused by a chromosomal abnormality; the individual has three chromosomes (trisomy) instead of the normal two for the pair designated number 21; usually accompanied by some degree of mental retardation.

Dysarthria: A condition characterized by slurred, uncoordinated, imprecise speech due to motor dysfunctions.

Dysfluency: A breakdown in the prosodic flow or fluency of speech.

Dysphonia: An unpleasant sounding voice; partial loss of voice.

Echolalia: Parrotlike ("echoing") repetition of what is heard.

Emergent Literacy: The first signs of abilities and knowledge with regard to written language; the period between birth and the time when children conventionally read and write.

Epiglottis: Shieldlike cartilage that closes off the larynx during swallowing. Located at the back of the tongue, it acts like a hinged lid to close over the opening into the larynx. When we swallow, the larynx rises and the epiglottis closes over the glottis (space between the vocal folds) so that food is directed into the esophagus.

Esophageal Speech: A process of communicating in which the 1aryngectomized individual must inject air into the esophagus and then must set tissue at the top of the esophagus into vibration by expelling the air from the esophagus (forcing air into the esophagus involves production of consonants that require oral production).

Esophagus: Tube leading from the throat to the stomach.

Etiology: Cause.

Expiration: Exhalation or breathing out.

Expressive Language: The ability to produce information (oral expression and writing); the ability to use language.

Expressive Skill: The ability to express oneself in the language of signs and finger spelling.

Expiration: Exhalation or breathing out.

External Ear (Outer Ear): Concave, funnel-like structure for receiving sound.

Facial Nerve: Cranial nerve number VII; its function is motor control of the facial muscles (loss of function could result in Bell's palsy); its function includes sensory control of the anterior two-thirds of the tongue and the soft palate as well.

Fast Mapping: Quick incidental learning.

Feeling Function: The expression or response to feelings and/or attitudes.

Fetal Alcohol Effects (FAE): The cognitive and behavioral characteristics associated with fetal alcohol syndrome (FAS) without the characteristic physical abnormalities.

Fetal Alcohol Syndrome (FAS): A syndrome resulting from maternal alcohol intake during pregnancy, characterized by altered facial features, developmental delays in language and cognition, and behavioral problems.

Figurative Language: The use of words in a creative way, rather than literal, to create an imaginative or emotional expression; these forms include metaphors, similes, idioms, and proverbs.

Finger Spelling: Use of the manual alphabet to form words and sentences (also called the Rochester Method or Visible English).

Fluency: The flow with which speech is produced.

Fluency Disorder: The abnormal flow of verbal expression characterized by impaired rate and rhythm, which may be accompanied by struggle behavior.

Form: A component of language that includes syntax, morphology, and phonology; those components that connect sounds or symbols with meaning; the structure and sound of language.

Form of Language: The phonologic, morphologic, and syntactic systems of language.

Free Morpheme: One that can stand alone; it can function as a word.

Fricative: A consonant produced by forcing the airstream through a small opening so that turbulence is produced, such as /s/, /z/, /ð/, or /θ/.

Functional: Having no known origin or cause.

Function of Language: The pragmatic system; the social aspect of language.

Glides: Sounds produced by allowing the breath stream to flow or "glide," rather than being stopped or constricted.

Glossopharyngeal: Cranial Nerve number IX; its function is motor control of the pharynx and sensory control of the pharynx and tongue.

Glottal: A sound produced by constricting the space between the vocal folds, /h/.

Glottis: Small opening between the vocal folds when the folds are adducted (closed).

Hard of Hearing: A loss of 35 to 69 dB, which makes the understanding of speech, through audition, difficult, but not impossible.

Hard-of-Hearing Child: One whose hearing impairment, whether permanent or fluctuating, adversely affects its educational performance.

Hard Palate: The roof of the mouth and the floor of the nose.

Hearing Impairment: A condition caused when sound waves are interrupted on their way to the brain or when the brain cannot interpret the sound waves.

Hematoma: A swelling filled with blood; these lesions usually result from trauma, usually vocal abuse or violent coughing that causes a little hemorrhage just under the covering membrane.

Hemiplegia: Paralysis of one side of the body.

Hertz (Hz): Unit of frequency.

Hypernasality: Speech characterized by an excessively nasal voice quality.

Hypertonic: Excessively tense muscles.

Hypoglossal: Cranial nerve number XII; its primary function is motor control of tongue movements.

Hyponasality: Speech that lacks sufficient nasal quality.

Hypotonic: Lacking muscle tone.

Imagining Function: A function of communication that places the speaker–listener in a creative or imaginary situation.

Incus (anvil): Middle bone of the middle ear.

Individuals with Disabilities Education Act (IDEA): Formerly known as Public Law, 94–142, the Education for All Handicapped Children's Act, and its amendments, its name since 1990.

Inferior: Bottom or lower part.

Informing Function: A communication act that includes sharing or exchanging information.

Inner Ear: That part of the ear in which mechanical energy becomes electrical energy through vibrations, which stimulate the end organ of hearing.

Innervates: Supplies nerves to a body structure; stimulation by way of nerves.

Inspiration: Inhalation or breathing out.

Instructional Decision-Making: A process whereby a professional who is familiar with research-based instructional practices can implement these practices and strategies while consistently monitoring for student mastery of outcomes.

Integrated Thematic Instruction: Method of delivery of instruction where units and lessons are planned around common themes across subject areas. Within these themes, specific outcomes and competencies are common and therefore developed across each of the classes and/or subject area.

Interpreting: In hearing terminology, a signed and finger-spelled presentation of another person's spoken communication.

IPA: International Phonetic Alphabet; a system representing speech sounds symbolically.

Keytalk: A specialized computer program created by Laura Myers, a Child Language Development Specialist, for youngsters with voice disorders and language problems. The computer program simultaneously displays and says each letter, then a word, and sentence, as the child types on the keyboard. When the child is finished, the computer reads the whole sentence.

Kinesics: Nonverbal communication; the visual signals sent with the body movements of gestures, facial expressions, and posture.

Labiodental: Speech sound made by bridging the lower lip close to, or in contact with, the upper teeth, /f/, /v/.

Language: An organized set of symbols used for communication.

Language Acquisition Device (LAD): A specialized language processor in the brain that is activated by specific linguistic input. This device is said to make language acquisition possible.

Language Disorder: The impairment or deviant development of comprehension and/or use of a spoken, written, and/or other symbol system; may involve: (1) form of language, (2) content of language, (3) function of language in any combination.

Laryngectomee: One who has had a laryngectomy.

Laryngectomy: Surgical removal of the larynx.

Laryngopharynx: Portion of pharynx behind the larynx.

Larynx: Primary organ of phonation; responsible for voice production; located at the upper end of the trachea and extremely sensitive to irritation; composed of cartilage and muscular frames.

Lateral: Sides or margins.

Learning Disability: A disorder in one or more of the basic psychological processes involved in understanding or in using spoken or written language that manifests itself in the areas of listening, thinking, writing, reading, spelling, or computing mathematics.

Linguadental: Place of articulation wherein the tongue tip is brought to the upper teeth. [θ], [ð].

Lingualveolar: Place of articulation wherein the place of constriction is the front of the tongue against to the gum (/t/, /d/, /s/, /z/, and /n/).

Linguapalatal: The place of articulation wherein constriction is caused by the tongue raised against the hard palate.

Lip Reading/Speech Reading: Understanding the oral language or speech of a person through observation of lip movement and facial expression.

Liquid: A speech sound made with less oral constriction than a fricative but more constriction than a glide (/l/, /r/).

Malignant: "Evil"; cancerous.

Malleus: First and largest bone in the middle ear.

Malocclusion: Faulty positioning of the teeth that may result in an underbite or an overbite; any deviation from a normal symmetrical relation of the two dental arches.

Mandible: The lower jaw.

Manner of Articulation: How a sound is produced, the degree or type of constriction (plosives, fricatives, affricates, glides, liquids, nasals).

Manual Communication Board (MCB): An individually designed aid that has no electronic or moving parts. An MCB can meet many, but not all, communication needs. Elements of an MCB include the vocabulary, representations (symbol) system, symbol and display size (black-and-white, two-inch), vocabulary arrangement (checkerboard, columns, solid), and organization (nouns, verbs, objects, situational).

Maxillae: The two bones that make up most of the hard palate. The upper jaw.

Mean Length of Utterance (MLU): A measure of syntactic development based on the average length of a child's sentences; scored on transcripts of spontaneous speech.

Mental Retardation: Significantly subaverage general intellectual functioning existing concurrently with deficits in adaptive behavior and manifested during the developmental period that adversely affects a child's educational performance.

Mesial/Medial: Midline.

Metalinguistic Awareness: The ability to reflect on language as a decontextualized object and to use language to talk about language.

Metaphor: Figure of speech in which one thing is called by the name of another to indicate the similarities between them, for example; "He's a rock of Gibraltar."

Microcephaly: Abnormal smallness of the head.

Micrognathia: Abnormal smallness of the jaw, especially the lower jaw.

Middle Ear: Part of the ear that directs sound energy to the oval window, via the ossicles.

Mills v. DC Board of Education: A decision passed in 1972 that required the District of Columbia to provide a free, appropriate public education for students with disabilities.

Modified Transistor Radio: This device serves as an audio oscillator signaling device that can be operated by a single external switch. A sound is emitted when a button is pressed that will let teachers or other communication partners know that the user has something to say or wants to amend something said earlier. Instructions for modifications and use are described in the operations manual, with suggestions for switch use and mounting.

Morpheme: The smallest unit of meaning in a language.

Morphology: The rules that govern the parts of words that form the elements of meanings and the structures of words; the rule system that governs the structure of words and word forms.

Mother–Infant Attachment: The strong affectional relationship between a mother and her infant; said to serve as the cornerstone for the social emotional development of young children.

Motor Nerve: A nerve that stimulates muscle contractions.

Multidisciplinary Team Approach: An approach utilized by a group of professionals from different disciplines to assess the individual needs of a child. Through communication and collaboration, the multidisciplinary team formulates recommendations of all aspects of the child's problems that fall within their area of expertise. Parents are an integral part of the multidisciplinary team.

Multimodal System: An approach that utilizes the individual's full communication capabilities, including any residual speech or vocalizations, gestures, signs, and aided communication.

Nares: The nostrils.

Nasals: sound produced by the breath stream passing through the nose (/m/, /n/, /ng/.

Nasopharynx: The portion of the pharynx behind the nose.

Obturator: A prosthetic appliance used to close an opening in the hard palate.

-ology: The study of.

Organic: Having an anatomic or physiological cause.

Organ of Corti: Sensory part of the cochlea that contains cells and rests on the basilar membrane.

Orofacial: Relating to the mouth and face.

Oropharynx: The portion of the pharynx behind the mouth.

Orthodontist: A dentist trained to align teeth and correct malocclusion.

Otitis Media: Inflammation of the middle ear.

Oto-: Relating to the ear.

Otolaryngologist: Ear, nose, and throat specialist; a member of the cleft palate interdisciplinary team.

Otosclerosis: Hardening of bones in the middle ear.

Paralanguage: Sounds produced in speech that are not part of the phonetic code.

Pathology: Disease, injury, or malfunction of a body part.

Pedodontist: A dentist who specializes in the dental care of children and works with a team in management of a child's dental care.

Pennsylvania Association of Retarded Children v. Pennsylvania Board of Education: A 1972 state decision that required the state of Pennsylvania to provide a free, appropriate public education for students with mental retardation.

Perinatal: Relating to the period just before or just after birth.

Personal Amplification: Devices, such as hearing aids and cochlear implants, that enhance sounds.

Pharynx: Upper throat cavity; primary organ of resonation; the throat.

Phonation: Generation of voice by means of a vibrating structure, usually the vocal folds.

Phoneme: Smallest unit of speech; each language has its own set of phonemes. In English, phonemes are identified according to their manner, place of articulation, and whether the sound is voiced or unvoiced.

Phonetics: Study of speech sounds, without regard to meaning. The study of the way speech sounds are articulated.

Phonics: The system by which symbols represent sounds in the alphabetic system.

Phonology: Study of speech sounds of language; the sound system of a language, including the rules that govern various sound combinations.

PL 94-142: A 1975 federal law that mandates that each child between the ages of three and twenty-one with a disability must be provided a free, appropriate public education in the least restrictive environment.

Place of Articulation: Where in the oral cavity the essential articulatory contact or movement is being made; the primary articulators that shape the sound (bilabial, labiodental, linguadental, lingualveolar, linguapalatal, linguavelar, glottal).

Plosive: A speech sound that is produced by completely stopping the air flow (/p/, /b/, /t/, /d/, /k/, and /g/).

Pneumatic Larynx: Primarily used by laryngectomees to help them talk, a device that is placed over the stoma in the neck through which the laryngectomee breathes.

Polyps: Any mass or tissue that bulges or projects outward or upward from the normal surface level. If a polyp appears on the vocal fold, it tends to interfere with contact between the folds during vibration. The result may be breathiness in the voice.

Posterior: Back.

Postnatal: Occurring after birth.

Prader-Willi syndrome: A chromosomal disorder characterized by muscular hypotonia, obesity, short stature, hypogonadism, and some degree of cognitive malfunction.

Pragmatics: Study of language in context; in part, focuses on the intention of the communication.

Prelingual Deafness: Loss of hearing occurring before the development of speech and language skills.

Prelinguistic: Skills that are prerequisite to language learning.

Premaxilla: Anterior and inner portion of the maxilla, further divided by a suture between the two incisor teeth on each side into two bones (center portion of gum); the front portion of the maxillary bone.

Prenatal: Preceding birth.

Presbycusis: Sensorineural hearing loss, due, in part, to old age.

Preverbal: Occurring before an infant can speak.

Prosody: The rhythm of speech, including rate and intonation.

Prosthesis: An appliance used to compensate for a missing or paralyzed structure.

Prosthetic Appliance: An appliance attached to one's body to replace or supplement the natural part, e.g., an obturator.

Prosthodontist: A medical doctor with a specialty in the construction and fitting of various dental appliances.

Proxemics: Distance in interpersonal communication.

Proximal: Toward the midline or center.

Psychogenic: A condition thought to be caused by underlying psychological or personality factors.

Psycholinguistic Theory: A linguistic approach to language acquisition that states that the human brain contains a mental plan or structure to understand and generate language and that the plan is guided by an independent rule system.

Receptive Language: The ability to understand language.

Resonance: Quality of sound created by vibrations in the vocal tract.

Respiratory System: Energy source for speech.

Rhythm: See **Fluency.**

Ritualizing Function: A communication act that includes the social amenities or customs within a specific culture such as greeting, apologizing, and regulating turn-taking in games or talking on the telephone.

Root: Back portion of the tongue.

Semantics: The study of meaning, or the system of features that structures a language's vocabulary.

Semicircular Canals: Three looped bony tubes located in planes at right angles to each other and opening into the vestibule; they enable an individual to maintain balance.

Sensorineural Hearing Loss: Hearing impairment resulting from a pathological condition of the inner ear along the nerve pathway from the inner ear to the brain stem.

Sensory Nerve: A nerve that conveys impulses from a sense organ to the central nervous system.

Serious Emotional Disturbance: A condition exhibiting one or more of the following characteristics over a long period of time and to a marked degree that adversely affects educational performance: for example, an inability to learn that cannot be explained by intellectual, sensory, or health factors; an inability to build or maintain satisfactory interpersonal relationships with peers or teachers; inappropriate types of behavior or feelings under normal circumstances; a generally pervasive mood of unhappiness or depression; or a tendency to develop physical symptoms or fears associated with personal or school problems" [Code of Federal Regulations, Title 34, 300.7(b)(9)].

Simile: An explicit comparison between two dissimilar things, for example, "He laughs like a hyena."

Social Interactionists/Sociolinguistic Theory: This theory views language within its social context. Social interaction and relationships are deemed crucial because they present the child with the framework for understanding and formulating linguistic content and form.

Spastic: The most common type of cerebral palsy, which results in tense, contracted muscles; also accompanied by persistent primitive reflexes, and absence or delay of normal motor skills.

Special Educator: A professional trained to work with learning and developmental needs of children with disabilities.

Speech: Audible production or representation of language. It is the result of manipulation of the vocal tract and the oral musculature.

Speech Disorder: Impairment of voice, articulation of speech sounds, and/or fluency.

Speech-Language Pathologist: An educational specialist concerned with identification, assessment, and treatment of problems of speech, language, and voice.

Speech-Language Pathology: The study of abnormalities of speech, language, and voice.

Spinalaccessory Nerve: Cranial nerve XI; its function is motor control of the shoulder, arm, and throat movements.

Stapes (stirrups): Third and smallest bone in the middle ear.

Stoma: In laryngectomees, the hole in the neck through which the person breathes after a laryngectomy.

Strategy: A specific way of using AAC aids, symbols, and/or techniques more effectively for enhanced communication. A strategy, whether taught to an individual or self-discovered, is a plan that can facilitate one's performance.

Stuttering: The involuntary repeated and prolongation of speech sounds and syllables.

Subaverage Intellectual Functioning: An IQ standard score of approximately 70 to 75 or below based on individually administered general intelligence tests that were designed for the specific purpose of assessing intellectual functioning.

Superior: Top or upper part.

Supraglottis: The part of the larynx below the vocal folds, but above the trachea.

Symbols and Symbol Systems: A visual, auditory, and/or tactile representation of conventional concepts (e.g., gestures, photographs, manual sign sets/systems, pictoideographs, printed words, objects, spoken words, Braille).

Syndrome: A group of symptoms that occur together.

Syntax: Linguistic rules governing the order and combination of words to form sentences and the relationships among the elements within a sentence.

Technique: A method of transmitting messages (linear scanning, row-column scanning, and encoding, signing, natural gesturing).

Thorax: The chest.

Thyroid Cartilage: Largest of the cartilages; often referred to as the "Adam's apple"; it forms an anterior wall for the larynx and protects its interior.

TMJ: The temporal mandibular joint; the joint that connects the mandible and maxilla.

Tourette Syndrome: A neurological disorder characterized by tics and involuntary rapid sudden movements that occur repeatedly in the same way.

Trachea: The windpipe.

Transverse: A horizontal cut at any level.

Trigeminal Nerve: Cranial nerve number V; its function is motor control of the jaw movements and sensory control of the face. This is the nerve into which dentists inject novocaine.

Tympanic Membrane: The eardrum.

Unaided: A technique that does not require any physical aids; manual, gestural, manual/visual, sign, or facial communication.

Unilateral Paralysis: A condition in which one of the vocal folds is paralyzed, resulting in aphonia.

Use: Pragmatics; the rules that govern language use in social contexts.

Uvula: The hanging portion of the soft palate; tip of the soft palate.

Unvoiced Sound: A speech sound that does not include vibration of the vocal folds.

Velopharyngeal: Pertaining to the soft palate and the posterior nasopharyngeal wall. Velopharyngeal closure is essential for many speech sounds and to separate the nose from the larynx during swallowing.

Velopharyngeal Closure: A process that occurs when the velum (soft palate) and pharyngeal walls act together to direct air and voice through the mouth rather than the nose.

Velopharyngeal Incompetence: The inability to achieve total closure of the nasal cavity during speech.

Velum: The soft palate.

Ventral: The belly.

Vocabulary Development: The acquisition of new words and new meanings and the establishment of links between them.

Vocal Folds: Source of voice; located on both sides of the larynx; The ligaments of the larynx. They stretch across the interior of the larynx and abduct (draw away from) and adduct (move toward).

Vocal Nodule: Buildup of a callouslike substance on the vocal fold.

Vocal Polyp: Tissue enlargement that may be filled with fluid or other matter.

Voice: Vibrations of the vocal folds.

Voice Disorder: Although there are varying definitions of what constitutes a voice disorder, most researchers agree that a voice disorder is one wherein quality, pitch, loudness, or flexibility differs from the voices of others of similar age, sex, and cultural group.

Voiced Sound: A sound produced by vibration of the vocal folds.

Voiceless Sound: A sound produced without vibration of the vocal folds.

Vowel: A sound produced with a relatively open vocal tract that allows for a continuous, unrestricted airflow. All vowel sounds are voiced.

Word Finding: The ability to store and retrieve words, thoughts, and a sequence of events.

Author Index

Subject Index